NARRATIVE MATTERS

A *Health Affairs* Reader

~

NARRATIVE MATTERS

The Power of the Personal Essay

in Health Policy

Edited by

FITZHUGH MULLAN, M.D.

ELLEN FICKLEN

and

KYNA RUBIN

Foreword by

ABRAHAM VERGHESE, M.D.

THE JOHNS HOPKINS UNIVERSITY PRESS

Baltimore

© 2006 The Johns Hopkins University Press
All rights reserved. Published 2006
Printed in the United States of America on acid-free paper
2 4 6 8 9 7 5 3 1

The Johns Hopkins University Press
2715 North Charles Street
Baltimore, Maryland 21218-4363
www.press.jhu.edu

Library of Congress Cataloging-in-Publication Data
Narrative matters : the power of the personal essay in health policy / edited by
Fitzhugh S. M. Mullan, Ellen Ficklen, and Kyna Rubin.
p.   cm.
"A *Health Affairs* reader."
Anthology of essays published in the Narrative matters section of Health affairs journal.
Includes bibliographical references and index.
ISBN 0-8018-8478-0 (hardcover : alk. paper) — ISBN 0-8018-8479-9 (pbk. : alk. paper)
1. Medical policy.   2. Narrative medicine.
[DNLM: 1. Health Policy—United States—Collected Works.   2. Delivery of Health
Care—United States—Collected Works.   3. Health Knowledge, Attitudes, Practice—United
States—Collected Works.   4. Medicine—United States—Collected Works.
5. Narration—United States—Collected Works.   6. Public Health—United States—
Collected Works. WA 540 AA1 N106 2006]   I. Mullan, Fitzhugh.   II. Ficklen, Ellen.
III. Rubin, Kyna.   IV. Health affairs (Project Hope)
RA393.N37 2006
362. 1—dc22
2006005257

A catalog record for this book is available from the British Library.

CONTENTS

FOREWORD

It is a pleasure to write a foreword to a unique collection of health policy narratives, the best of the best. I have watched the *Narrative Matters* section of *Health Affairs* evolve from a novel, almost experimental section conceived by Fitzhugh Mullan and John Iglehart in 1999, to its present status where it seems to have always been part of *Health Affairs*.

When the editors announced this new section of *Health Affairs*, I was delighted—here was yet another outlet for the stories that are so much a part of our professional and personal lives. But I wondered if it would survive. When the time came for budget cuts and pruning of pages, would the qualitative nature of such a section make it an instant target, the first to be sacrificed?

Even if I had doubts about its longevity, I loved the title of this new section—*Narrative Matters*. Yes, it does. I would have been tempted to use an exclamation point: Narrative Matters! But then the word play around the other sense of this phrase—matters that relate to narrative—would have been lost. The title was more than clever; it was audacious and it was contrarian. In a health care world where money talks, where the income from an invasive cardiology section might underwrite the activities of an entire medical school department, where medical-industrial complexes were merging to create "economies of scale," the editors of *Health Affairs* were holding up something different from the quantitative, evidence-based articles that occupy most of their pages; they were showcasing narrative and, by doing so, putting a human face on the policy issues discussed in the rest of the journal.

Times have changed, and we seem to live in a medical world much more willing to concede that stories are important. I have been privileged to give grand rounds occasionally on literary matters, things quite apart from and yet having everything to do with clinical medicine, the sorts of things that would have been unlikely topics for grand rounds just fifteen years ago. The whole business of story and narrative was viewed as "soft" by leaders in the medical and health policy communities. I remember one well-known chair of a department of medicine who was introduced to me minutes before I was to give grand rounds to his department. He was alarmed that I had no slide carousel, no thumb drive with my PowerPoint files. His anxious reaction only added to my stage jitters, but I was committed. I told stories. I read passages of prose. It went well. Afterward, the house staff wanted to continue a dialogue that I did not know I had begun. Story had engaged their right brains as only story will do. Story had let me connect with some essential part of them. I had no PowerPoint, but I had story.

The reflective essays found in *Narrative Matters* represent a movement in the health policy world that is seen elsewhere in both medicine and the general public. Writing is hugely popular. Op-ed pages and features are an increasingly important part of print journalism. The *New England Journal of Medicine* recently started publishing personal reflections, and *JAMA* has published "A Piece of My Mind" section for some time. It is as if a nutrient whose absence had caused a deficiency has suddenly been restored to the drinking water.

I celebrate such writing and the impulse to write, the impulse to share some transformative incident that I am privileged to have witnessed. In my own writing, I often feel that I write in order to understand what I am thinking. Mysteriously, insight comes (when it does come) in the very *act* of writing, as if only by sitting with pen and pad can we snatch it out of the ether.

The essays in this collection embody another aspect of writing: the writer captures a unique and personal experience that in its uniqueness is also archetypal. We marvel at a tale so foreign to our experience, but at another level we identify with it completely. With the best of such writing, we walk away feeling that we have been given *two* gifts: instructions for living, and a sense that we are not alone.

Health affairs—not the journal, but the state of the country's health system—are in a mess. The world of academic health centers, where I work, is a rich one full of rewards, trials, and great discoveries, but also contrasts, inconsistencies, and inequities. The doctor's world, as rewarding as it is, is also a world of secrecy and loneliness—no one can fully walk in our shoes. We guard our patients' secrets and we witness their suffering. We know better than any that death can come so unexpectedly, so unfairly; yet subconsciously we believe some contract we have made with the fates gives us immunity. Perhaps related to this, or perhaps related to more global stress and responsibility, we find dysphoria and depression are all too common in our profession. Anyone who doubts this has only to look at the alarming statistics on physician suicide and drug addiction to know that it is true.

I mention this because I think that at one level the impulse to write—not only for doctors but also for patients, family members, and others—is also the impulse to sort out our feelings, to bring about a healing, by which I mean simply a coming to terms with ourselves or our environment. Even when writing can't change the root causes of our malaise (an aging population, rising health care costs, decreasing reimbursement, nonphysicians dictating how much time doctors spend with patients), what it can do is acknowledge the disquiet. "What Are We Going to Do with Dad?," for example, is the title of one powerful essay in this collection. The essay form can tackle the big themes: suffering, poverty, aging, and death. But it can also capture the small satisfactions that mean nothing, but mean everything and that can save us. I like to think it is what physician-poet William Carlos Williams was getting at when he wrote:

> *so much depends*
> *upon*
>
> *a red wheel*
> *barrow*
>
> *glazed with rain*
> *water*
>
> *beside the white*
> *chickens.*

Williams was ahead of his time, depicting in his essays and poems both the euphoria and the dysphoria of doctoring. It was an experience uniquely his, unique to Paterson, New Jersey, and the era in which he lived. But in the very act of trying to describe it, trying to give it form on the back of a prescription pad while sitting in his car, or clacking away at his typewriter late at night, he was also dealing with it, processing it, paring it down to its lowest common denominator so that years later a reader would say, "Yes, that is exactly how it feels." I think Williams would have approved of this collection. Narrative, he would have said, matters.

Abraham Verghese, M.D.
Joaquin Cigarroa Jr. Chair and Marvin Forland Distinguished Professor
Director, Center for Medical Humanities and Ethics
University of Texas Health Sciences Center, San Antonio

PREFACE: ABOUT THIS BOOK

If a picture is worth a thousand words, a good story is worth many columns of statistics. Stories present ideas, conflicts, and, sometimes, resolution. They have depth and dimension, drama and emotion, making them more memorable than data alone.

This belief in the power of the story encouraged us—with support from the Kellogg Foundation—to start the Narrative Matters section of *Health Affairs* in 1999. It seemed to us that the personal narrative could bring a perspective to the quantitative material traditionally published in the journal that would promote understanding and help focus policy deliberations. In this spirit, one of us (John Iglehart*) wrote the following in the Editor's Note in the first issue that carried Narrative Matters in July 1999:

> In the eighteen years that Project HOPE has published *Health Affairs*, America's medical care system and the making of health policy have become big business. But the voices of patients, their families, and their caregivers have often gotten lost in the relentless shuffle. *Health Affairs* is a policy journal, and I never regarded publishing material that emphasizes the personal, the subjective, and the autobiographical as its reason for being. But through a confluence of factors, I have come to believe that we could enrich the journal by nurturing a form of health policy writing that affords greater opportunity for new voices to contribute to future debates.

As we embarked on this adventure, we were aware of precedents in the field. Susan Sontag, tackling cancer in *Illness as Metaphor*, and Samuel Shem, writing with biting humor about the dehumanizing of medical education in *House of God*, would not have counted themselves as policy writers but were important contributors to the conversation in health policy at the time. More recently, Abraham Verghese and Atul Gawande, writing in the *New Yorker* and elsewhere, have used

---

*John Iglehart is the founding editor of *Health Affairs*.

their own experiences to raise understanding and concern about health policy issues—from AIDS in Appalachia to errors at the operating table. Fictionalized health policy narratives arrive in our living rooms nightly, with shows like *M*A*S*H* and *E.R.* raising awareness and affecting opinions about all manner of health issues from battlefield medicine to the health care safety net. *Academic Medicine,* the *Annals of Internal Medicine,* and the *Journal of the American Medical Association* have their own literary sections that bring a human dimension to their pages.

Our enthusiasm for the narrative form was tempered by knowing that storytelling is not science but perception. As such, it is vulnerable to all of the human hazards of subjectivity. Dan Fox famously said that the plural of anecdote is policy, suggesting the force of the narrative. Harvey Fineberg noted, admonitorily, that the repetition of anecdote is not evidence, reminding us of the challenges that await the policy narrative editor. We have taken this concern seriously, using both the editorial staff of *Health Affairs* and a wide range of peer reviewers to read and critique every manuscript submitted. Although this does not exempt the column from subjectivity, we have invoked a process that brings many eyes and much thoughtful criticism to every published manuscript.

The column has been popular from the outset with both readers and writers. Readers often tell us that the Narrative Matters section is the first one they turn to when opening the journal. There is brisk business in hits and downloads for Narrative Matters articles on the *Health Affairs* Web site. The U.S. Office of Civil Rights, the *Washington Post,* the *Los Angeles Times,* and National Public Radio have featured Narrative Matters writings and authors. Narrative Matters writers have come from many walks of life, including patients, the parents and children of patients, physicians, nurses, politicians, and foundation executives. Topics, likewise, have ranged widely, including essays on AIDS, drugs, death, race, old age, wheelchairs, drunk driving, and kidney transplants.

The popularity of Narrative Matters as a policy forum as well as the wonderful literary renderings of many of the essays generated the idea of an anthology—an idea with which the Johns Hopkins University Press concurred. In selecting forty-six essays from among the more than eighty published to date, we chose those we believe to be very well written on representative subjects that remain topical—although this latter criterion did not present much of a problem because so many of the policy issues in health care seem to live forever. To help the reader select essays of particular interest we organized the essays around themes that reflect ongoing policy struggles.

We hope that putting these articles back into play in the form of an anthology allows them to continue to contribute to the policy debate in the United States. Many of the essays raise issues of principle and ethics about U.S. health care that will need to be addressed by people on the street as well as by health professionals and policymakers if health care cost, quality, and equity are to be improved. We hope that the book will be used by citizens and policymakers not only as a good read but also as a staple of their libraries. Policy narrative has an important role, as well, in the curriculum of future health care leaders. We hope, therefore, that this anthology finds its way into the curriculum in schools of medicine and public health and in programs on bioethics, the medical humanities, public policy, and political science. Finally, we hope that the writings in this volume will stimulate others to reflect on their own lives and write health policy narratives that increase the level of understanding and promote health improvements.

From the outset, our partner in Narrative Matters has been the W. K. Kellogg Foundation. It supported the Narrative Matters section in *Health Affairs* from its inception and has provided additional funds for conferences, evaluation, and planning this volume. We think that the Narrative Matters idea is consistent with the values of the Kellogg Foundation, which include community participation, outreach, and the democratization of health care. Special acknowledgment and thanks go to members of the Kellogg Foundation staff, including Gloria Smith, Pat Babcock, Barbara Sabol, Marguerite Johnson, and Alice Warner-Melhorn.

At *Health Affairs*, Andrea Zuercher, Sue Driesen, and Meredith Zimmerman helped ready the essays for original publication. We also thank Michael Stein for his work preparing the anthology for publication and Donald E. Metz, the journal's executive editor, for his unwavering encouragement. At the Johns Hopkins University Press, Wendy Harris and Carol Zimmerman calmly guided us through the book publication process.

We hope that you read the following essays with interest and feel encouraged to write health policy narratives of your own. *Health Affairs* would like to keep an active flow of essays so that policymakers never lose sight of the human consequences of policy decisions, both in the United States and around the world.

Fitzhugh Mullan, M.D.
Ellen Ficklen
Kyna Rubin
John K. Iglehart

CONTRIBUTORS

BARRY ADAMS, a registered nurse, is a doctoral student at Brandeis University's Heller School of Social Policy in Waltham, Massachusetts, where he is studying work, inequality, and social change. His dissertation will focus on nurses and their work.

ANDREW BATAVIA was an associate professor of health law and policy at Florida International University (FIU) in Miami, Florida. He was associate director of the White House Domestic Policy Council under President George H. W. Bush and a former legislative assistant to Sen. John McCain (R-AZ). Batavia, who died in 2003, was posthumously awarded full professorship and tenure at FIU.

RAY BINGHAM is a registered nurse certified in neonatal intensive care who has written about his nursing experiences in the *American Journal of Nursing* and the *Washington Post*. He is a technical writer for the National Institute of Nursing Research at the National Institutes of Health in Bethesda, Maryland.

W. RICHARD BOYTE is an associate professor of pediatrics in the Department of Pediatrics at the University of Mississippi Medical Center in Jackson.

HOWARD BRODY is a professor of family practice and also works in the Center for Ethics and Humanities in the Life Sciences at Michigan State University in East Lansing.

NEIL CALMAN is a practicing family physician and president of the Institute for Urban Family Health in New York City.

DAVID CARLINER is cofounder of Elder Health, based in Baltimore, Maryland. The organization operates special needs Medicare Advantage programs and prescription drug plans in Maryland, Delaware, the District of Columbia, Pennsylvania, and Texas. It also helped major Medicare Advantage providers in ten states identify people eligible for both Medicare and Medicaid. Carliner is a partner at the Shelter Group, where he oversees the growth of the organization's senior housing division.

DANIEL DERKSEN is a professor in the Department of Family and Community Medicine at the University of New Mexico School of Medicine in Albuquerque. He is director of the UNM Center for Community Partnerships and principal investigator for the W. K. Kellogg Foundation's Community Voices initiative to improve health care services and access for uninsured and underserved populations in eight New Mexico counties.

RHIANNON TUDOR EDWARDS is a senior research fellow in health economics and founding director of the Centre for Economics and Policy in Health at the University of Wales, Bangor, in the United Kingdom.

VANESSA NORTHINGTON GAMBLE is director of the Tuskegee University National Center for Bioethics in Research and Health Care in Tuskegee, Alabama.

RICHARD GARCIA is a pediatrician in Stockton, California. He is working on a documentary on U.S. health disparities and a collection of essays on race in American medicine.

JANET GILSDORF is a professor of pediatrics and director of pediatric infectious diseases at the University of Michigan Medical School and a professor of epidemiology at the University of Michigan School of Public Health in Ann Arbor. She also directs the *H. influenzae* Research Laboratory and the Cell and Molecular Biology in Pediatrics Training Program.

MARTHE GOLD is the Logan Professor of Community Health and Social Medicine at the City University of New York Medical School. A family physician, she was senior policy adviser in the Office of the Assistant Secretary for Health, U.S. Department of Health and Human Services, from 1990 to 1996. She directed the Panel on Cost-Effectiveness in Health and Medicine, whose final report is used in academic and policy settings.

MAHLON JOHNSON is a professor of neuropathology at the University of Tennessee Graduate School of Medicine and is on the staff of the University of Tennessee Medical Center in Knoxville, Tennessee. He is the author of *Working on a Miracle* (Bantam Books, 1997).

PAUL JUNG completed training as a Robert Wood Johnson Clinical Scholar at the Johns Hopkins University. He is currently an officer in the Commissioned Corps of the U.S. Public Health Service, based in Washington, D.C.

ALOK KHORANA, a graduate of Maharaja Sayajirao University (India), is an assistant professor of medicine at the James P. Wilmot Cancer Center and the Department of Medicine, University of Rochester (New York).

JANETTE KURIE is director of behavioral medicine for the Pennsylvania State University/Good Samaritan Hospital Family and Community Medicine Residency Program in University Park. She is a former member of the Pennsylvania Attorney General's Family Violence Task Force and that state's Child Fatality Review Committee.

SHARON LADUKE has been a registered nurse for more than twenty years, working in acute care, education, human resources, and information management. She is the manager of a medical-surgical unit in a community hospital and writes about nurses' experiences with the legal system.

RICHARD LAMM is director of the Center for Public Policy and Contemporary Issues at the University of Denver (Colorado). He was governor of Colorado from 1975 to 1987.

JOHN LANTOS is chief of general pediatrics and associate director of the MacLean Center for Clinical Medical Ethics at the University of Chicago (Illinois). His books include *Do We Still Need Doctors?* (Routledge, 1997); *The Lazarus Case: Life and Death Issues in Neonatal Intensive Care* (Johns Hopkins University Press, 2001); and *Neonatal Bioethics: The Moral Challenges of Medical Innovation* (Johns Hopkins University Press, 2006).

DAVID LAWRENCE retired in December 2002 after eleven years as chairman and CEO of Kaiser Foundation Health Plan and Kaiser Foundation Hospitals in Oakland, California. He is the author of *From Chaos to Care: The Promise of Team-Based Medicine* (Perseus Publishing, 2002).

MICHAEL LERNER is president and cofounder of Commonweal, a health and environmental research institute in Bolinas, California, and of the Smith Farm Center for the Healing Arts in Washington, D.C. He is also president of the Jenifer Altman Foundation and the Barbara Smith Fund and cofounder of the Health and Environmental Funders Network.

CAROL LEVINE is director of the Families and Health Care Project at the United Hospital Fund of New York.

JOHN McDONOUGH is executive director of Health Care For All in Boston, Massachusetts, and former health committee chairman in the Massachusetts House of

Representatives. He is the author of *Experiencing Politics: A Legislator's Stories of Government and Health Care* (University of California Press and Milbank Memorial Fund, 2000).

FITZHUGH MULLAN is the Murdock Head Professor of Medicine and Health Policy at the George Washington University and a staff physician at the Upper Cardozo Community Health Center in Washington, D.C. He is a contributing editor to *Health Affairs* and editor of the Narrative Matters section.

DANIELLE OFRI practices and teaches medicine at Bellevue Hospital/New York University School of Medicine. She is editor-in-chief and cofounder of the *Bellevue Literary Review*. Her writing has appeared in *Best American Essays, Best American Science Writing*, the *New England Journal of Medicine*, and the *New York Times* and on National Public Radio. Ofri is the author of two collections of essays, *Singular Intimacies: Becoming a Doctor at Bellevue* (Beacon Press, 2003) and *Incidental Findings: Lessons from My Patients in the Art of Medicine* (Beacon Press, 2005).

PAUL RAEBURN, a former editor and writer at *Business Week* magazine, is the author of *Acquainted with the Night: A Parent's Quest to Understand Depression and Bipolar Disorder in His Children* (Broadway Books, 2004).

KAREN ROBERTS is a nurse practitioner and writer in Lawrence, Kansas. She works for the Internal Medicine Group.

MICHAEL ROWE is an associate clinical professor in the Yale School of Medicine's department of psychiatry and codirector of the Yale Program on Recovery and Community Health in New Haven, Connecticut. He writes about homelessness, mental illness and community mental health services, and doctor-patient relationships, among other topics. He is the author of *The Book of Jesse* (Francis Press, 2002).

BARBARA SHARF is a professor of communication at Texas A&M University in College Station, Texas.

DAVID STEINBERG is director of the Section of Medical Ethics at the Lahey Clinic Medical Center in Burlington, Massachusetts. He is editor of the *Lahey Clinic Medical Ethics Journal* and an assistant clinical professor of medicine at Harvard Medical School.

DEBORAH STONE is a research professor of government at Dartmouth College in Hanover, New Hampshire. She writes on health insurance, disability, and care-giving and is the author of *Policy Paradox: The Art of Political Decision Making* (W. W. Norton, 2001).

LISA SWEETINGHAM is a staff writer for *Court TV* online (CourtTV.com), where she covers national news on crime, courts, and the justice system. She currently lives in Los Angeles.

SHARON TERRY is president and CEO of the Genetic Alliance (a coalition of advocacy organizations in Washington, D.C.) and founding executive director of PXE International (an advocacy organization for the genetic condition pseudo-xanthoma elasticum, PXE). She is an adviser to the National Institutes of Health, Centers for Disease Control, U.S. Food and Drug Administration, and various nonprofit groups.

IRENE WIELAWSKI is a freelance health care journalist and editor in Pound Ridge, New York, who formerly was on the staff of the *Los Angeles Times*.

DARRYL WILLIAMS is director of the Office of Border Health at the Texas Tech University Health Sciences Center at El Paso. He was principal investigator for the W. K. Kellogg Foundation's Community Partnerships in Graduate Medical and Nursing Education in El Paso. The program created a consortium of local hospitals and universities that together operate four clinics in isolated rural communities in El Paso County, including the clinic in San Elizario portrayed in his essay.

JERALD WINAKUR has practiced internal medicine and geriatrics in San Antonio, Texas, for almost thirty years. His essays, fiction, and poetry have been published in numerous journals, and for many years he was a contributing editor of *Mediphors: A Literary Journal of the Health Professions*. He is an associate faculty member at the Center for Medical Humanities and Ethics at the University of Texas Health Science Center in San Antonio and a lecturer in humanities at the University of Texas at San Antonio.

ABIGAIL ZUGER is an infectious disease specialist in New York City. She writes frequently on medical issues for the *New York Times*. She is the author of *Strong Shadows: Scenes from an Inner City AIDS Clinic* (W. H. Freeman, 1995).

NARRATIVE MATTERS

CHAPTER 1

WRITING TO CHANGE THINGS

ESSAYS ON THE POLICY NARRATIVE

Me and the System: The Personal Essay and Health Policy
FITZHUGH MULLAN

Using and Misusing Anecdote in Policy Making
JOHN E. McDONOUGH

Out of the Closet and into the Legislature: Breast Cancer Stories
BARBARA F. SHARF

～ Me and the System

The Personal Essay and Health Policy

*Writing is an invitation to change things, to battle mortality, and
to connect the little picture with the big.*

FITZHUGH MULLAN

Back in 1972, when I first set about recording my experiences as a "rad-
ical" medical student at the University of Chicago and as a resident
in the Bronx, a fellow activist challenged me. "Where do you come
off writing your memoirs?" she asked with an in-your-faceness characteristic
of the time. "Who do you think you are, anyway? Fidel or somebody?" I
struggled with that one. What egotistical urge had driven me to write? Was
it vanity or was it hubris? I am sure that there was a bit of arrogance underlying the desire to tell my story—as there has to be for anyone recording a
memoir. If, after all, the memoirist doesn't think he or she has an important
tale to tell, there is little likelihood of persuading anyone else of its significance. But the sentiments that prompted me and others to write in the first
person go well beyond the venal and the self-promotional.

I wrote, first of all, because I thought I had lived through events that were
worth recounting—big events and small ones. I had marched with Martin
Luther King Jr. in Chicago shortly before his death and had been "liberated"
by Puerto Rican militants, the Young Lords, when they took over Lincoln
Hospital in the Bronx a few years later. I had campaigned on behalf of a class-
mate against a medical school policy that required him to shave his beard
on pain of expulsion; and I had felt a man's bowels grow cold after a failed
emergency operation to stem the flow of blood from his ruptured aorta. I
wanted to tell about these things because they were important to me and because I thought that they would speak to other people as well. For me and,
I believe, for others, generous instincts—the urge to record, to share, and to

explain—are at the heart of the personal essay. "I was there; you should have seen it" are sentiments that drive the memoirist. I wanted people to know what had happened in the Civil Rights movement, in medical school, and in some very tough hospitals in the Bronx. I wanted what I had lived through to make sense to them. Chastened but not deterred by my colleague's reproach, I went on to write a book called *White Coat, Clenched Fist: The Political Education of an American Physician*, a long personal essay about those earlier years.

Goading Those in Charge

Had someone asked then if I was writing about health policy or to affect health policy, I probably would have said no. Yes, I was writing to inform people, to persuade them of the need for reforms, but I didn't see myself as delivering a blueprint for change; nor did I see myself talking to the politicians and policymakers per se. I was describing what I had seen in the hope that someone might listen and join in an effort to make things better. And yet my belief was that what I had experienced was representative of what went on elsewhere and that it should be of interest to people outside of my immediate world. In retrospect, I was indeed writing to influence policy. I was telling stories that were pertinent to people's concerns about health care and that were, to some degree, a goad to those in charge. My writing was an invitation to change things.

In the years since *White Coat*, I have continued to write on a regular basis—commentaries, health policy articles, book reviews, and history. Time and again, though, I have returned to the genre of that first volume, the personal essay. Sometimes in short columns and sometimes at book length, these essays have drawn on my own life to document and dramatize the quandaries and opportunities inherent in our system of health care. I have come to believe that the first-person narrative is an important art form in health care and a potential player in the making of policy.

A second reason I write personal essays is common, I think, to many people who write: the battle against mortality. Writing makes a record, a mark on the world, no matter how small. One's written words become one's offspring. The stories and their messages will live on as evidence of one's presence on the planet and engagement with life. This instinct calls on people to write about their work. Although best known as a poet, William Carlos

Williams left an eloquent record of personal essays about his work as a general practitioner in Paterson, New Jersey, during the middle years of the twentieth century. Lewis Thomas wrote regularly in the *New England Journal of Medicine* and elsewhere about his life as a physician, a scientist, and an administrator. Along the way, he published an essay called "Illness," which reflects on his experience as a patient. Indeed, sickness reminds us most aggressively of our mortality and inspires many to put pen to paper. In *Heading Home,* a powerful narrative about the importance of his personal life, Paul Tsongas wrote movingly of his newly diagnosed cancer and his decision to leave the U.S. Senate in 1984—a farewell that proved to be a premature sign-off to his public career. Don Cohodes, a senior policymaker at the Blue Cross and Blue Shield Association for many years, described his battle with terminal cancer in "Through the Looking Glass: Decision Making and Chemotherapy" (*Health Affairs,* Winter 1995), arguing persuasively that heroic measures were good for the doctor but not for the patient.

In 1975 I was found to have a mass in my mediastinum, the area above the heart and between the lungs. Even before the obligatory biopsy was undertaken that proved it to be cancer, I had begun to contemplate writing about what was happening to me. I believe that I buffered myself against fear and uncertainty by considering that I was some sort of journalist about to undertake an assignment in a dangerous land—and report back about it. The "trip" took more than two years and was truly awful. Although my desire to write disappeared completely during that time, it returned when my health improved: *Vital Signs: A Young Doctor's Struggle with Cancer* appeared in 1983, followed by a *New England Journal of Medicine* piece called "The Seasons of Survival: Reflections of a Physician with Cancer." These essays (one long and one short) said to me and to the world that I wasn't dead and that I had perspectives on cancer and cancer care learned from my painful journey that might be of use to other people.

Commentaries such as those of Williams, Thomas, Tsongas, Cohodes, and myself offer the personal essayist a voice in life's ongoing debates, an epistolary vote in the ultimate making of policy by people usually removed in time and space from the writer's personal struggle. That vote and the influence it can carry is an important currency for the personal essayist. It is substantive and permanent. It is a little bit of immortality.

A third reason that I write is a conscious urge to connect my little picture with the big picture. This may not move all personal essayists, but it moti-

vates me and is at the core of why the personal essay can speak with eloquence to broad issues of common concern. The link between what I experience personally and the forces that govern society frequently seems quite
real to me. For instance, what I perceived as the social myopia and the implicit racism that were part of my medical education troubled me, but these
were also issues for society as a whole and for medical educators in particular. More recently, after many years away from patient care while I served as
an administrator and a policymaker in the U.S. Public Health Service, I re-
trained in pediatrics and went back to work at an inner-city clinic in Washington, D.C. This was like getting out of the sky suite and back into the ball
game after many years as a general manager. It was exciting and rejuvenat-
ing. It was a throwback and it was a new world. A surprising number of things
hadn't changed—the patients, the shortcomings of the inner-city system, the
satisfaction of practice. Many things, of course, had changed quite a bit, including the numbers of new medications and the advent of managed care.

Being back in practice has given me much to write about that connects
my daily experiences with the larger world of health policy and with the very
issues with which I struggled as a federal policymaker for many years—care
for the uninsured, medical education policy, and public health practice. So
now I am a practitioner once again as well as a veteran of the land of policy.
The essayist in me cries out for the one world to talk to the other, so I have
been writing a series of commentaries based on my clinical work for the
Washington Post under the title "From the Clinic." These pieces are not
health policy proposals in any finite sense but are written with an eye to a
readership populated with politicians and policymakers.

The personal essay as a policy piece has a strong tradition in medicine.
Atul Gawande, writing "When Doctors Make Mistakes" this year in the *New
Yorker,* and David Hilfiker, writing "Facing Our Mistakes" in the *New England Journal of Medicine* some years ago, raise the difficult and troubling
issues about physicians' shortcomings as seen in their own practices. The
eloquence of these candid reflections and the fact that this is an area about
which few physicians write combine to make these narratives classics. Abraham Verghese has earned literary accolades for his autobiographical writings
that intertwine his medical work and his personal life. In his first book, *My
Own Country: A Doctor's Story,* Verghese serves as the reader's guide on a
tour of human immunodeficiency virus (HIV) as it arrived in rural America.
Over and over again, that tour invites the reader to consider his own re-

sponses to acquired immunodeficiency virus syndrome (AIDS), both as an individual and as a member of society. Verghese's story brims with health policy implications. Robert Coles has practiced what might be called the "personal documentary" as a variant on the personal essay in his Pulitzer Prize–winning *Children in Crisis* series. Coles uses a documentary approach to depicting children in various settings but remains a prominent presence throughout the accounts; his surmises about the children and their problems are not lost on the reader.

Natural as it might seem as an art form, the writing of personal narrative is not without hazards. Its very spontaneity can be a problem. To work, the essay must be an intimate document in which the writer shares observations and thoughts with candor. Yet our own spontaneous inner voices do not always make good copy. They can wander, suffer from mean-spiritedness or naïveté, groan under the load of ego, or arrive on the page as trivial despite our previous belief that they were visionary. This problem is compounded because the personal essayist writes not only about himself but about other people. The essayist must find a voice that is candid enough to sustain the personal quality but is simultaneously fair to others involved in the story— patients, spouses, family, and colleagues. Calibrating the role of the "I" in the first person is difficult as well. First-person narratives are effective because the reader wants to see inside the life of another person, to compare lots, to identify with or, on occasion, reject being identified with the writer. Yet "I" and "me" can easily become oppressive, turning the reader off and undercutting both the art and the import of the piece. The best first-person essays are unobtrusively first person, creating a comfortable atmosphere for the reader where the message of the narrative is not obscured by the personality of the messenger.

The Power of Anecdote

Writing about one's own experience is an exercise in subjectivity. The very power of the personal essay comes from the view of the world as seen through the eyes of the writer, who is unapologetically the arbiter of fact and significance in the narrative. The circumstances reported and the valence they are given are the sole and unchallenged domain of the writer. Anecdote, attitude, prejudice, and point of view are prominent and important components of the personal essay. Although personal observation holds a time-honored place in the history of science, the subjective characteristics of the personal essay are not prominent values in the science of today, nor are they part of the growing efforts in the field of health policy to make decisions based on quantitative measures. Terms such as "evidence-based" and "data-driven" are the coin of the policy world today, and "the anecdote" as evidence is as much demeaned in policy circles as it is in clinical medicine. Yet, important as the arguments are for the use of quantitative science to inform clinical and policy decisions, the anecdote—the report of life events from an unabashedly subjective vantage point—remains a powerful tool for focusing the human mind. The historian and health policy commentator Dan Fox is fond of saying that, for better or worse, "The plural of anecdote is policy." The "Harry and Louise" anti–Health Security Act television ads of 1994 are potent examples of the use of anecdote (out of context, synthetic, and dramatized, to be sure) to sway public opinion about health policy. Vignettes about health maintenance organizations (HMOs) in the movie *As Good as It Gets* and conflicts over HIV disclosure policy in the television drama *ER* often engage public attention on health policy issues more effectively (this is not to say, more accurately) than the pronouncements of learned commissions, op-ed pieces, and health policy journals.

The question, then, may well be asked about the appropriateness of the personal narrative, with its cargo of subjectivity, in a health policy journal. Health care—giving it, getting it, administrating it, teaching it—is a realm of human enterprise that is often personal, frequently dramatic, and always laced with controversy. It is a rich domain for chroniclers who draw on the personal and the subjective—fiction writers, TV producers, and cinematographers—as well as for the writer of the first-person narrative. The personal narrative is indisputably a compelling vehicle for transporting perspective and opinion about health policy issues. The first-person essay, in fact, can lend perspective and vitality to issues that are appropriately and simultaneously being explored and written about in a quantitative and analytic fashion. Personal reflections can add dimension and depth that will make the issue both more lucid and more interesting. The challenge for a journal whose principal product is analytic and not literary is to find writers who can steer their way between the hazards of ego and introspection on the one hand and pure editorializing on the other. The use of peers (providers, patients, ad-

ministrators, and teachers) to review submissions will do a great deal to re-
fine the selection process and to protect against the potential excesses of style
or point of view.

Human beings have always had stories—and always will. Health (and
health policy) is a quintessentially human realm, and its stories are as vivid
and revealing as those from any area of human endeavor. Even as we move
to put decision making in health on a firmer, more quantitative basis, our
stories can help to maintain perspective and promote wisdom. That is the
mission of Narrative Matters.

⌒ Using and Misusing Anecdote
in Policy Making

*A former state legislator explains the beauty and peril of allowing
storytelling into the policy process.*

JOHN E. McDONOUGH

In 1991 I was a legislator in the Massachusetts House of Representatives
arguing against deregulation and market-based health care as a means
of controlling health care costs. I carried a nine-inch pile of evidence
everywhere—to hearings, press conferences, meetings, and floor debate.
Half the pile was made up of empirical, peer-reviewed studies demonstrating the efficacy of state-run hospital rate-setting programs. The other half
consisted of peer-reviewed studies failing to identify improvements in cost or
access from managed care. By contrast, deregulation advocates—corporate
benefit managers, insurance and hospital executives, and union welfare
fund trustees—had no empirical evidence to support their case.

My opponents were unimpressed by my pile and, in the context of the
times, were right. They knew what they saw on the ground—a bewildering
regulatory behemoth, calcified by years of political deals between hospitals

Volume 20, Number 1: 207–212. January/February 2001.

and the state, that prevented them from negotiating contracts that would give them more value and accountability. My studies were based on pre-1985 data; the research community pretty much gave up studying rate setting after that, satisfied with results showing that it worked. But the fast-changing health system bore little resemblance to that earlier period, and the research community had yet to grasp what was happening in the field. My adversaries spoke from the real world, telling anecdotes describing their actual experiences in controlling costs by becoming active, aggressive purchasers of health care. In the end, their perspective mattered more than the reams of scientific evidence I brought to the debate.

The lesson that personal observation can easily trump hard data revealed itself again to me the following year. I lacked firsthand knowledge of the 1993 bill mandating Massachusetts insurers to pay for bone marrow transplants for breast cancer patients because I didn't sit on the relevant committees. But I had read accounts of the hearings and discerned a familiar dynamic. Breast cancer victims and their advocates argued that greedy insurance companies and HMOs refused to pay for these transplants, regardless of the benefits, because they were too costly. Women who had undergone this treatment testified to its life-saving value. Insurers argued that the treatment's efficacy had not been scientifically demonstrated and that suffering from the treatment was as inordinate as its cost. They were then portrayed as callous, white, male-dominated parties who were insensitive to women's health needs.

When a Story Is Off Base

I considered taking issue with the bill but had learned, as most legislators do, to pick my fights. Initiating opposition that would be futile and would be viewed as blind to women's health needs didn't make sense. The measure passed both houses easily and was signed into law by then Gov. William Weld, an otherwise vigorous critic of health insurance mandates. A similar pattern played out in many other states and the federal government, which approved their own mandates in the 1990s.

But the rush by providers, patients, and states to provide, obtain, and finance these services had an unfortunate effect. Researchers could find few volunteers for controlled studies to evaluate the treatment's effectiveness. Indeed, not until 1999 were studies completed demonstrating that bone marrow transplant, much more costly and painful than conventional treatments, was no more effective in extending the lives of breast cancer victims.

These two encounters illustrate both the value and the harm of relying on storytelling in making public policy. Stories can enable lawmakers to understand a legitimate need for policy change but can, just as readily, lead them to make bad policy decisions. Stories can bring to life drab data analyses, helping us to visualize problems and opportunities for change. But stories also can lead us down wasteful and dangerous paths and blind us to uncomfortable truths that we would prefer to ignore, like the fact that there is yet no easy cure for breast cancer.

It comes as no surprise, then, that almost as common as using narrative and anecdote in policy making is criticizing them. Former Minnesota state legislator Lee Greenfield often remarks that one compelling anecdote (true or false) at a crucial moment in a floor debate can vaporize a mountain of data and careful policy analysis.

Anecdote's Inescapable Humanity

Why is narrative so central to policy making? Because it is central to life. We live our lives crafting, telling, and receiving stories. We tell our loved ones stories from our day. We catch up with old friends by sharing tales from our lives. We receive, from all forms of the media, stories to help make sense of our world. In constructing our stories, we are necessarily selective in choosing and editing details to drive home a lesson; to engage our audience; or to meet time, space, and other constraints.

This is true for the hardest of sciences. "So much of science proceeds by telling stories," writes Harvard naturalist Stephen Jay Gould in *Bully for Brontosaurus: Reflections in Natural History*. He sees us as "vulnerable to the constraints of this medium" because we are unaware of our tale telling in observing the natural world. "We think that we are reading nature by applying rules of logic and laws of matter to our observations," he says, "but we are often telling stories."

Policymakers, like scientists, are as human as the rest of us. Part of our uniquely human heritage involves telling stories to find meaning from the events, data, and stimuli in our lives. Most policymakers, and especially legislators, have not had training in research methods and thus share the layperson's suspicion of statistical analysis. The adage "Lies, damn lies, and statistics" makes more sense to most of them than does the value of the r-square.

Values versus Data

Perhaps the real power of stories lies in their reflection of ideas and values. As Deborah Stone argues in her book *Policy Paradox*, much of the policy process involves debates about values masquerading as debates about facts and data. "The essence of policymaking in political communities [is] the struggle over ideas," she writes, even though in legislatures and other deliberative bodies, participants engage in fierce debate about data and statistics as though the process were a straightforward search for truth. Her view, which I share, challenges the concept of policy making as simply a scientific exercise in data analysis.

I recall numerous debates in the Massachusetts legislature on whether to mandate use of seat belts and motorcycle helmets, provide clean needles to addicts, require insurance coverage for infertility treatments, dictate gun ownership restrictions, and obligate employers to provide health insurance to their workers. In each case, both sides argued about data as if identifying the right statistic would compel the other side to surrender. But data were only rhetorical weapons used to bolster competing values.

When policy differences are grounded in divergent value structures, empirical research rarely helps much until participants allow for those value differences. Recognizing the differing value frameworks marbled through a policy dispute can enable participants to reach a resolution that acknowledges those differing concerns or can make it clearer why agreement is not possible.

In 1995, while I was chairman of the legislature's insurance committee, I remember how community housing activists fought with insurance company executives over home insurance "redlining"—an unwillingness to write coverage of homes in marginal urban neighborhoods. A series of trust-building exercises brought both sides to a greater appreciation of each other's differences and led to passage of consensus anti-redlining legislation the following year.

That said, stories' power also can have an adverse effect. When false or out-of-context stories provide the basis for public policies that impose requirements on unwilling citizens, those suffering the imposition may, with reason, feel indignant. An untrue or misused story in everyday life holds little impact beyond a few individuals, but in public policy it may result in adverse consequences for millions. Ronald Reagan's reference to a mythical Chicago welfare queen — happily collecting her monthly check while sitting pretty at home — tarnished the way Americans viewed recipients of government assistance in ways that set the tone for a public and congressional backlash against helping needy populations in the early 1980s.

Using Stories Wisely

The question to ask is, How do we craft a more appropriate role for narrative and anecdote in the policy process? Narrative should be to policy making what suitable case study is to empirical research. Case study alone can never establish scientifically based claims but does play a key role in the research enterprise. One valid, well-documented case study can effectively demolish a theory, demand rethinking of an approach, or set the stage for further empirically based investigations.

In a similar way, contextually appropriate stories used in the policy environment can identify important, neglected policy problems. For example, no policy analysis can illustrate the need for culturally competent health care as compellingly as Anne Fadiman's account of a Hmong child's experience with epilepsy in *The Spirit Catches You and You Fall Down*. Anecdotes help to signal problems with existing programs or policies that have been unrecognized or insufficiently understood. They can even provide evidence that a program or law is working as intended. Stories assist policymakers in thinking about the consequences of rival policy choices. Also, most policy decisions cannot wait for the gold-standard randomized clinical trial, and many others do not even lend themselves to scientific investigation. Valid stories and anecdotes are better than nothing to guide decisionmakers. Stories also help policymakers to think about the potential political impact of their policy decisions.

Stories even benefit lawmakers when the going gets tough. In my years in the Massachusetts legislature, I developed great affection and respect for the long-serving representatives who would regale newer members with tales from other eras. During the difficult fiscal crisis of 1989–1991, hearing their stories of what worked to control the impact of the previous fiscal meltdown (in the mid-1970s)—and understanding that "this, too, shall pass"—was enormously helpful when the pressures seemed unending.

But using narrative to make policy requires the same standards of validity as those applied to case study. Lack of accountability is the bane of storytelling in the policy environment. A story needs to be true and presented in a context that does not distort its relevance to the policy choice at hand. Red herrings are unacceptable. For instance, I remember that to prove their harmlessness, an angry landlord once ate lead paint chips before a Massachusetts legislative health committee hearing. Policymakers must develop the necessary discipline to be intelligent consumers of anecdotes.

How Do You Know That?

Given the pace and frenzy of their world, policy veterans may find it unrealistic to consistently pay scrupulous attention to sources and truth. The most valuable approach may therefore be a defensive one. A research methods instructor taught me that one of the most powerful questions one can ask is, "How do you know that?" After receiving his advice, I began asking this question carefully and respectfully in public hearings and in corridor conversations. I was amazed by the results. The most brazen and self-confident witness could melt when pressed for the validity and appropriateness of a source. A few choice responses: "I read it somewhere, but I can't remember where." "My brother told me." "Everyone knows that!" (my personal favorite).

Asking "How do you know that?" may not come naturally to policymakers. Many public officials develop (or possess *a priori*) a tendency to accept the individual stories of their constituents. Perhaps they do this in response to routine accusations of losing contact with the "folks back home." Real folks don't discuss the latest issue of the *New England Journal of Medicine*; they tell stories about their lives. And when they meet a politician, they continue their storytelling to communicate what's important to them.

Some constituents' stories are off the wall, while others are pertinent and valuable. The challenge is not to get narrative and storytelling out of policy making. They are oxygen to the process and cannot be eliminated. We might as well try to ban conversation. The challenge is to raise everyone's skill level—officials and citizens alike—to be more intelligent consumers of stories.

~ Out of the Closet and into the Legislature

Breast Cancer Stories

How narratives about one disease have shaped policy.

BARBARA F. SHARF

Twenty-three figures appear in living color in photographs before and after breast cancer surgery in *Show Me*, a recent book in both print and online forms. The women display in stark detail lumpectomies, mastectomies, and reconstructions, along with their individual reactions to these treatments. Clearly, women have come a long way since the stigmatized silence of twenty years ago, when poet and cancer sufferer Audre Lorde urged them to "become visible to each other" in order to "translate the silence surrounding breast cancer into language and action." Her statement was considered revolutionary because, with few exceptions, women then did not disclose their personal stories of breast cancer to one another privately, let alone publicly. Yet by the 1990s the walls of silence had crumbled, and personal narratives of living with breast cancer became nearly ubiquitous — through conversations, popular books, newspapers and magazines, television, and Internet chat rooms.

Personal stories of breast cancer have raised social awareness, destigmatized the disease, and been key in creating significant changes in health policies. Legislative allocations, medical standards of care, and scientific research priorities have all been altered by women's storytelling about breast cancer. Shifts in policy influenced by powerful illness narratives have been mainly positive, but sometimes compelling stories can lead to undesirable outcomes as well.

Volume 20, Number 1: 213–218. January/February 2001. The study discussed in this essay was partially funded through U.S. Department of the Army Grant no. DAMD17-97-1-7240.

One-Breasted Women on the Steps of Congress

Audre Lorde wonders in *The Cancer Journals,* "What would happen if an army of one-breasted women descended upon Congress?" Lorde presaged the notion that women with breast cancer can join together to influence the policy-making process. She alerted us to the idea that shared biographies are integral to advocacy; and advocacy, of course, can alter policy.

Indeed, in the words of Rose Kushner, "It helps to be stubborn and have a loud voice." Even before Lorde's vision of women with breast cancer descending upon Washington, another woman's foresight had brought change to medical practice. In 1975 Kushner, a journalist and cancer survivor, put her investigative skills to use in understanding the life-threatening disease that afflicted her. *Breast Cancer: A Personal History and an Investigative Report* was a brief account of her own illness, with a lengthy analysis and critique of the then current epidemiological and clinical approaches to breast cancer. Kushner called for women to participate in making their health care decisions in an informed manner. Her book was excerpted in newspapers and women's magazines, and remained in circulation until the early 1990s. With instincts far ahead of her time, Kushner brought to the surface a number of policy-related issues still debated today, including environmental toxins, the limits of mammography in detecting cancer, the dangers of irradiation, and the need (or not) to undergo mutilating surgery.

Kushner's most direct impact on policy involved the question of why it was standard medical procedure for physicians to perform a one-step biopsy and mastectomy. Patients were routinely expected to give consent to this procedure before anesthesia, thus facing the terrifying prospect of waking up to find a confirmed diagnosis of cancer and their breast gone—all in one fell swoop. Kushner found a well-qualified physician who agreed to a two-step process for her that separated biopsy results from surgical treatment. This gave her a chance to rebound from the bad news about her biopsy result and consider her options. Her subsequent research supported her argument that a two-step process would benefit women psychologically while not harming their prognosis. Based on this information and her own tenacity, Kushner single-handedly lobbied the cancer establishment to change the customary treatment, which had been based on tradition and paternalism rather than evidence. Her efforts resulted in a change of standard clinical procedure to the two-step biopsy and treatment decision — an amazing feat for a lone citizen-activist. Fortunately, today's Rose Kushners needn't act alone.

The Multiplying Effect of Numbers

"We start today's program with a moment of silence for Marian Cortez [not her real name] who died April 3 of this year, two months from her fiftieth birthday . . . Her passion for finding a cure for this disease to save her daughter from its ravages was as great as her compassion for those afflicted with it." Thus opened a plenary session at a National Breast Cancer Coalition (NBCC) advocacy training conference in 1999.

The NBCC, formed in 1991, now comprises more than 500 groups and 60,000 individuals. Its mission is to promote research; improve access to screening and treatment, especially for the underserved and uninsured; and increase survivors' influence in creating and implementing legislation, regulation, and clinical trials. For the past nine years the group has sponsored an annual advocacy training conference, attended by hundreds. Participants are provided information on new medications, research initiatives, and legislative process to enable them to speak with credibility about the legislative priorities identified by NBCC. (In 1999 priorities included increased funding for peer-reviewed research, follow-up treatment for women found through federal screening programs to have cancer, and insurance coverage of treatment for people participating in clinical trials.) The beginning of each half-day session is marked by a tribute to a deceased person remembered for her efforts in breast cancer advocacy. These remembrances take the form of a mini-narrative of the person's life and contributions as her image is shown on wide-screen monitors. The memorials are poignant, reminding each participant of her own mortality, underscoring the importance of the day's activities, and vividly illustrating the direct link between health legislation and individual lives. The conference culminates in Lobby Day, when participants noisily demonstrate outside Congress, then organize by state to talk with their elected representatives about the NBCC's prioritized issues.

When Cancer Hits Home

On the other side of the equation, legislators can be especially receptive to cancer narratives when they or someone they love has had cancer, or when constituents convey cancer stories. Two examples spanning both sides of the political aisle in Congress underscore the power of health narratives to affect political agenda setting.

Sen. Tom Harkin (D-IA) has championed funding of various medical research projects throughout his lengthy career. Breast cancer has been his central focus over the past decade. Harkin — a senior member of the Senate Appropriations Subcommittee on Labor, Health and Human Services, and Education — characterizes cancer as "a leading killer." His interest in the disease is also influenced by the fact that according to his office, "his only two sisters died at a young age from breast cancer. Neither of them had ever had a mammogram, and if they had, he strongly believes they would be alive today." His legislative achievements include dramatically increasing funding of breast cancer research and creating treatment, prevention, and screening programs for lower-income women.

Members of Congress don't have to be personally involved with the disease to be moved by cancer stories. Former Sen. Alfonse D'Amato (R-NY) had also been a member of the Senate Appropriations Committee. To my knowledge, D'Amato did not face a personal or close familial encounter with cancer as did Harkin, but he was swayed by the stories of a large number of Long Island constituent-survivors who suspect an environmental link to the cancer cluster in their community. The senator's motivation may have begun as a political move to procure women's votes, but D'Amato became a valuable ally to several local advocacy groups and to the NBCC.

Making Bad Policy

Personal accounts of illness can create a huge stir but may not always result in positive consequences. One case in point is the story of Nelene Fox, a thirty-eight-year-old California mother of three. In 1993, after being diagnosed with advanced breast cancer and exhausting all conventional therapies, she was advised by her doctors that her only remaining chance for survival was an autologous bone marrow transplant (ABMT), a risky process involving extremely high doses of chemotherapy. Her HMO refused to pay for the $140,000 procedure because the treatment was classified as "experimental," meaning that insufficient scientific evidence existed to prove that it extended a patient's life. Fox's local community raised the money for treatment, but she died soon after it.

Sympathizers speculated that she was unable to begin treatment in time to get the beneficial effect. Her brother, a lawyer, sued the HMO and convinced the jury to award $89,000 in damages to her family. Similar lawsuits with similar results soon followed. Questions that many physicians had about the efficacy of ABMT were compounded by prolonged difficulty in recruiting enough subjects for controlled clinical trials, since patients with advanced disease were repeatedly told at cancer centers that this treatment had shown promise. Media publicity about the Fox case succeeded in forcing widespread insurance reimbursement, further discouraging patients from enrolling in clinical trials. Thus, conclusions about the efficacy of the treatment were tragically delayed until 1999, when the National Cancer Institute announced that, based on available studies, ABMT does not benefit persons with breast cancer.

The Nelene Fox story and others like it persisted for nearly a decade. For years women fought to have ABMT, even though there was little or no data to support this choice. As John McDonough notes in the previous essay, going this route meant that the evidence that can only come from clinical trials was tragically delayed. In the end, we have come to discover that the insurers had valid grounds for their decision to withhold payment and that we held on to a story of false hope for much too long.

Personal breast cancer stories have inspired efforts by citizen-advocates and legislators to provide better care and more resources for the disease. But as the ABMT experience makes painfully clear, individual stories should not be taken as scientific proof.

Moving Beyond the Disease-of-the-Week

Breast cancer stories' influence on policy also raises larger, more difficult questions about how the national health care budget should be determined, as each disease-specific group organizes to ask for more attention and increased funding. Breast cancer advocates in the 1990s adopted the successful strategies of AIDS activists in the previous decade. Breast cancer advocacy, in turn, is informing efforts to focus on ovarian and prostate cancers, and the list of disease advocacy groups continues to grow. NBCC leaders argue that we should increase the total budgetary pot for health care so that all problems are adequately addressed, but this solution seems hopelessly unrealistic. Prevention, for example, continues to be shortchanged, despite the fact that national health care spending is already at an all-time high.

Narratives about disease invariably lead to the question of how we decide which disease deserves the most notice. Should disease incidence rather than visibility be emphasized as a more important criterion for policy concern? If so, then heart disease, which hasn't generated as many moving stories as have AIDS and breast cancer, should be our nation's central focus. The public and Congress have heard most about AIDS and cancer because of the vocal strength of those constituents. But heart disease, the biggest killer in this country, affects far greater numbers: More than 500,000 women die from cardiovascular disease each year, compared with 43,000 from breast cancer. Yet the National Institutes of Health budget to research heart disease is half a billion dollars less than that for AIDS, which ranks seventeenth among diseases causing mortality in the United States. Do heart disease advocates need to create more affecting personal illness stories? It seems inevitable that the squeaky-wheel-gets-the-grease approach to appropriations will pit one worthy group against another, or that attention will pivot from one priority to the next before long-term outcomes can occur.

Personal narratives are powerful rhetorical strategies as well as humane expressions of suffering and memorials to loved ones. The riveting communication of such narratives enlightens our understanding of what it means to live with breast cancer (or Alzheimer's or Parkinson's or spinal cord injury). As a society, however, we need to develop more sophisticated criteria for evaluating illness narratives. This is a knotty task because stories of suffering have authenticity and validity both for the teller and for fellow sufferers. In using personal narratives to affect health policy, the challenge is to effectively combine the emotional *pathos* and character-related *ethos* of stories with the other form of rhetorical proof, *logos* (the rational). Recipients of illness stories—be they lawmakers, policy wonks, or the public—face difficult questions. What are the criteria for making judgments about stories as a basis for generalizing public policy? How do we distinguish among competing narratives when all are compelling? Is it possible to move to a different level of storytelling, one that transcends competing narratives? The value of grappling with such complex questions is self-evident to those of us who remember an era when women didn't tell breast cancer stories.

CHAPTER 2

DOLLARS AND SENSE

HARD FINANCIAL REALITIES

Gouging the Medically Uninsured

A Tale of Two Bills

A health journalist encounters the gap between what providers charge insured patients and what they charge the uninsured.

IRENE M. WIELAWSKI

Not long ago my son had surgery to repair four small hernias. They were lined up in a row, extending vertically above his navel. Like so many of the weird things teenage boys come home with, this one left his father and me scratching our heads and, when the drama was over, very grateful for health insurance.

Andrew is a budding Ska trombonist, playing a style of music that combines reggae and rock. He had just played his first club gig with a band of high school boys whose performance style calls for energetic dancing while playing horns, drums, guitars, and keyboard as loudly as possible. Andrew gave it his all and, literally, the surgeon told us later, came close to blowing his guts out.

Hernia repair is a routine surgical procedure, and so it was for Andrew. Only after he recovered did we come to appreciate the edge insurance had given us in negotiating the health care system and how differently the system responds to patients without insurance.

Underlying this divide is a Byzantine pricing structure that reflects widespread discounting for patients with insurance, while obscuring the actual value of health services. Health professionals exasperatedly roll their eyes when asked to explain it. "Crazy." "Government in action." "A paperwork nightmare," they say. Less recognized are the inequities this pricing system imposes on those least able to bear up: the medically uninsured. These pa-

Volume 19, Number 5: 180–185. September/October 2000. Based in part on material gathered during the author's six-year evaluation of Reach Out: Physicians' Initiative to Expand Care to Underserved Americans, a grass-roots health reform program sponsored by the Robert Wood Johnson Foundation.

tients are being charged as much as twice what the rest of us pay for exactly the same medical service.

Pricing Run Amok

I would not have paid as close attention to the routine insurance company missives that filled our mailbox in the weeks after Andrew's surgery had I not, some months earlier, met Frederick Paquette, a sixty-two-year-old uninsured carpenter in Sacramento, California, who also needed hernia surgery. I had interviewed Paquette in my capacity as a medical journalist, tracking a grassroots health reform experiment.

The hardship of being uninsured and having to pay out of pocket for medical treatment is an old story. But since the failure of national health reform, Congress and the Clinton administration have all but abandoned the uninsured, even as their numbers creep steadily upward, rising 40 percent in the past decade to 44.3 million people.

But the current pricing situation, in which those least able to pay are being charged the most, gives the story a cynical new twist. Overcharging the uninsured is one of the many unintended and largely overlooked results of our decade-long obsession with curbing health care costs. Powerful interest groups — government, employers, insurers, hospitals, medical equipment vendors, and health care professionals — have fought vigorously to protect their interests. The uninsured, with no organized voice, emerge as losers.

Health care pricing is famously inconsistent. Urban versus rural, north versus south, slums versus hilltop — each has a different pricing structure. The situation brings to mind one of those houses jerry-rigged with additions to accommodate the space needs of a growing family. The result is, well, space. Unfortunately, the bathrooms are nowhere near the bedrooms, the kitchen is blocked off from the dining room, and Junior has to climb out a window to practice his curve ball against the garage. Space, yes, but in a completely illogical framework for family life.

So goes the tortured history of modern health care pricing, where the true value of any service is hidden behind walls of outdated federal regulation, complex reimbursement formulas, and discounts driven by the competitive marketplace of the 1990s. "It's like one of those things that just grows and grows and gets adjusted and modified here and there until it is so complicated no one even knows where to begin to fix it," a seasoned hospital executive told me.

Ironically, it was Medicare—the nation's first effort to improve access to health care for a vulnerable population—that launched the price inflation so discouraging to today's working poor. In rolling out this first national insurance program for the elderly in 1965, the federal government understandably did not want to negotiate with each and every doctor and hospital in the country. So it promulgated a series of rules that tied Medicare payments to a percentage of the average charge in a community or a percentage of the provider's own average charges, whichever was lower. If Doctor X, Hospital Y, and Laboratory Z had lower charges than the community average, Medicare's payment formula was a wake-up call to providers to start charging more so that they could get higher Medicare reimbursements. But to make a persuasive case, providers had to raise charges for all patients, not just the elderly.

Medicaid, the government insurance program for the very poor, added another pricing equation to the mix. Unlike Medicare, Medicaid is administered by individual states, which set fees early on according to whatever their legislatures decided to commit from the treasury. Today, states diverge widely in their reimbursements for identical medical services. Poorer states generally pay less, and, within each state, Medicaid generally pays less than Medicare.

To compensate for discounts to Medicare and Medicaid, providers once again sought refuge in inflated charges. This time privately insured patients were the target. In the 1970s and 1980s most private patients had indemnity insurance plans that typically paid 80 percent of full charges, with the patient responsible for the remaining 20 percent. By inflating charges to these insurers, providers were able to use the surplus they collected to offset losses from Medicare and Medicaid as well as for charity care to uninsured patients. Health care managers called it their "Robin Hood" gambit—a means of rationalizing the income stream even as quoted prices diverged evermore sharply from the true cost of doing business. The practice, known as cost shifting, prevailed for nearly two decades. Then private employers got wise to their role in balancing the health care ledger books, and they revolted.

The call to arms was a series of double-digit increases in the cost of employee health benefits during the late 1980s. Companies seeking to account for these premium hikes discovered that they were paying almost a third above the actual cost of medical care for their workers. They demanded relief. In the managed care revolution that ensued, they got it. The cross-subsidy was squeezed out. Insurance premiums stabilized. And a rash of consolidations and mergers in the managed care industry made new savings possible. As purchasers of services for large blocs of patients, insurers were able to extract their own discounts from health care providers.

The Rub

The depth of these discounts came home to me personally in the form of EOB (explanation of benefit) statements sent by our insurance company for Andrew's hernia surgery. Because I happened to be tracking Frederick Paquette's hernia case at the time, it was impossible for me to miss the contrast.

A pediatrician in our medical group saw Andrew the same day I called. The pediatrician thought that the small, soft lumps in Andrew's upper abdomen were hernias but wanted a surgeon's opinion. That appointment came a week later. In less than a minute of poking around, the surgeon confirmed epigastric hernias and conveniently scheduled surgery for the next school vacation. Andrew had a smooth recovery and was back to horn playing, baseball, and all the rest within a month. Besides the part of the insurance premium deducted from my husband's paycheck, the hernias cost us $30—representing copays for physician fees that are required by our managed care plan with Aetna U.S. Healthcare.

Aetna then proceeded to extract its discounts from Andrew's providers. To wit, the surgeon had billed $2,682 for his services; Aetna paid him $1,392. Our suburban New York hospital charged $2,593 for use of the surgical suite; Aetna paid $2,075. The pediatrician's $70 bill was knocked down to $37.25. Lab tests and an x-ray billed at $117 got discounted to $5.25.

Frederick Paquette, meanwhile, was making the rounds of Sacramento's surgeons and hospitals to see about getting his groin hernia repaired. Unlike Andrew, he did not have a referral, having depended upon low-cost public clinics for routine ailments. So right off, he encountered a cool reception that plummeted straight to the bottom line when he disclosed his lack of insurance.

Paquette was quoted full charges even though Sacramento is one of the most deeply discounted managed care markets in the country. Health plans there typically pay $3,000–$3,500 for comprehensive hernia care, including all physician fees and hospital charges. But to Paquette, surgeons quoted charges of $3,000–$5,000 for their services alone—a price range that would double when hospital charges were added. He had hoped to find a doctor willing to let him pay over time. But front-office staff brusquely insisted on a cash down payment. For hernia repair, it was $1,500.

At the time, Paquette and his wife had about $100 in savings. With no hope of raising the down payment, Paquette instead rigged himself with homemade trusses. His plan was to wait three years until he turned sixty-five and qualified for Medicare.

But the hernia worsened over the next year. Little by little Paquette gave up his carpentry jobs because lifting things hurt too much. Finally he reached a point where even walking was painful. That's when his luck changed, thanks to a charity project in Sacramento called SPIRIT, through which volunteer surgeons repair hernias for free and under whose auspices I met Paquette. Within a few weeks of the operation, he was free from pain and back at work—a testament to the simplicity of the fix both he and Andrew needed from our health care system but which only Andrew got in a timely and caring fashion. Had the SPIRIT project not existed, Paquette might eventually have staggered into an emergency room with a dangerously strangulated bowel at far greater cost to himself and the system than a reasonably priced hernia repair.

A Shameful Comparison

Arguably, Paquette might have found even reasonable prices discouraging. After all, he only had $100 in the bank, and no one seriously entertained his idea of paying for the surgery in installments. But when I look at the price discounts my son received from his providers and compare them with the lousy deals offered Frederick Paquette, my strongest emotion is shame. The pricing formulas that health care insiders deride as a "paperwork nightmare" are more personally punitive to the millions of people without insurance. A joint survey in 1997 by the Henry J. Kaiser Family Foundation and the Commonwealth Fund found that prohibitive cost led 55 percent of the uninsured to postpone care as Paquette did, 30 percent to skip treatment entirely, and 24 percent to not fill prescriptions—all of which can lead to far more complicated and costly illness. And the situation is worsening. The gap in drug prices alone for people with and without health insurance nearly doubled between 1996 and 1999, according to a government study.

I have not met anyone in health care who defends the current system of pricing. Most agree that it just happened and that no one intended for the uninsured to be charged more than everyone else. But people I talked to in my effort to reconcile Andrew's experience with Paquette's surprised me with arguments for the status quo.

The first argument was based on the millions of dollars in uncollectible bills that hospitals and other providers write off every year. Health care pricing is irrelevant, goes this argument, because the uninsured don't pay their bills. But many do. Next to the "uncollectable" column is usually one listing revenue from "self-pay" patients. And price absolutely influences purchasing decisions when the funds are coming out of your own pocket. For people living on very little, the decision to take an ailing child to the doctor can turn on the difference between $70 (the charge posted by Andrew's pediatrician) and $37.50 (the fee negotiated by our insurer).

The second argument was that the uninsured should negotiate their own discounts. Indeed, nothing in law prevents this. I have a friend who asks for discounts all the time, although financial hardship is not his motivation. As a medical malpractice attorney he knows the game so well that he doesn't need an insurance company to do his wrangling. For the unexpected disaster, he carries a major medical policy with a high deductible. For the rest, he offers to pay his doctors in cash whatever they get from insurers—no paperwork, no reimbursement delays. Few refuse the deal.

My attorney friend has little in common with the typical uninsured patient. He has the information, contacts, professional skills, and capital to make the pricing system work in his favor. Imagine Frederick Paquette trying to undertake such negotiations with the surgeons in Sacramento. He couldn't even interest them in an installment plan at full price.

Universal health insurance—in which everyone shared in the discounts—would solve this problem for the uninsured. But who can wait for that? Let's face it. The most recent universal coverage attempt, President Clinton's proposed Health Security Act, failed in 1994, and no political leader since has dared to renew the call. Incremental health reform seems to be the route our nation has chosen, and that has led to some noteworthy accomplishments. People can change jobs without losing their insurance, preexisting health conditions are less of a barrier to coverage, and more children are eligible for government-sponsored insurance. Now let's take a look at health care pricing and see if we can't come up with a way to protect the one in six Americans who lack insurance from being gouged.

Tea, Biscuits, and Health Care Prioritizing

An American visiting England observes initiatives to elicit public input on thorny health care allocation decisions.

MARTHE R. GOLD

It is mid-afternoon in December in a community meeting room in Wolverhampton, a small city in England's Midlands. It is damp and the wind is up, and it is nice to learn that afternoon tea will be served prior to conducting business. Daphne Austin, a public health physician from a local service agency, sets about serving tea and biscuits to nine people who have been recruited to discuss their views about National Health Service (NHS) coverage of an expensive new therapy. Since 1991, British government policy has mandated public involvement in health services decisions. Using a range of techniques for informed public involvement—polling, focus groups, and citizen juries in community and academic settings—the country has been developing methods for holding conversations with the public and feeding them back to the health care system. All of these techniques rely on deliberation—giving the public the tools and time to consider the pros and cons of various issues.

The people assembled today are middle-aged and older—three women and six men, all but one white. They are a convenience sample drawn from a citizens group that has agreed to consult when public input is deemed important to decision making in local venues. The Wolverhampton meeting is one of four, each with a different demographic makeup, that will advise the West Midlands Health Authority. Today's question is whether the thirty primary care trusts that are responsible for channeling funds and providing health care to the West Midlands region's 5.3 million people should extend coverage for enzyme replacement therapy to people suffering from Fabry's disease, Gaucher's disease, and other forms of Mucopolysaccharoidosis I.

I am in England on sabbatical, wearing the cloak of ambivalent advocate for the use of cost-effectiveness analysis to propel more equitable distribution of U.S. health care resources. My work in federal policy arenas has persuaded me that universal health care will come about only through rational and judicious use of health services. My work as a family physician and experience as friend and family member, however, have made me sensitive to the notion that utilitarianism in medical care has some fundamental difficulties. This is not an unrecognized issue in the policy literature back home, but in the United Kingdom explicit conversations about rationing on the basis of cost-effectiveness are being held in wide-open spaces. I am interested in seeing what regular Britons have to say about this. My notion has been that in a country with a global health care budget and relatively low (by Western standards) per capita investment in health care, the public must be more inured to the notion of rationing, or "prioritization," as it is often called here.

Painful Decisions

Shirley McIver, a Birmingham University expert in processes of public involvement in health care decision making, convenes the meeting. She introduces its intent: understanding how those present view the funding of a promising but expensive therapy for a rare disease. She asks participants to complete a questionnaire on their ideas about how much is reasonable to spend on any one person, and under what circumstances (to save a life or to treat a rare condition) spending thresholds should increase. After the surveys are filled out, McIver invites those assembled to openly discuss their answers. I am surprised, yet not surprised, to hear most of the participants say that the NHS should provide treatment regardless of cost. One middle-aged woman says, "They can find the money for wars, my darling, can't they?" Another says, "At the end of the day, there's nothing so precious as your relatives. Nothing so precious as love." A retired civil servant, however, sees things differently. He notes that there is "only so much money and you can't do everything."

Next, McIver tells the group about a rare inheritable condition that is known to affect 400 of the 52 million people served by the NHS in England and Wales. The condition has differing types and levels of morbidity that can affect the kidneys, heart, and brain. The group learns that before the development of a treatment (dubbed "Tdx" to cover a range of available enzyme replacement therapies), clinical management was aimed at relieving symptoms: dialysis for people with renal failure, medication and surgery for people with heart failure. According to McIver, treatment with Tdx is likely to allow early-treated people to live normal lives and diminish the chances of premature death for many. She cautions, however, that although evidence suggests that Tdx treatment is promising, it is a new therapy, and questions remain about the consistency of benefit across individuals and the drug's long-term effectiveness.

McIver then turns to the issue of cost. A year's treatment for children will cost about £125,000 ($225,000) and for adults about £350,000 ($630,000). Once started, treatment will generally continue for the rest of a person's life. McIver puts these costs into context by telling the group that the average spent by the NHS in a person's lifetime is £90,000 ($162,000) and the median, £40,000 ($72,000). Everyone finds this staggering; there is no doubt in the room that Tdx requires a new level of financial commitment. McIver tells the group that the drug is expensive because the company that makes it has to recover its development costs; that because only a few people will benefit from an "orphan" drug, development costs per patient treated are particularly high; and that a profit margin is added to this. She says that after a ten-year period of exclusive production, orphan drug status lapses and prices should fall, but by what amount is uncertain.

McIver reminds the group that finite budgets within the NHS mean that allocating resources in one place means rationing elsewhere. She asks about fairness: Is it right to disadvantage people with costly diseases because their condition takes a disproportionate share of care away from larger numbers of people with less costly conditions? She asks that the group also consider the precedent set by funding this therapy should a future expensive therapy come along for a different illness.

A Sticky Wicket

The group response is spirited and somewhat untethered. Irritation is near-universal at the government for underfunding health care. One older man complains, "There are two bloody doctors for 636 Members of Parliament," inveighing at the injustice of this, given the shortages and queues everyone else faces. Someone says that foreign visitors come to use U.K. health services for free, and a few people question whether there should be full health coverage for "asylum seekers," a.k.a. new immigrants. Another suggests that people with self-inflicted illnesses should not have their care paid for. Talk turns to George Best, the fallen Manchester United soccer hero who has received liver transplantation secondary to hepatic failure on the basis of alcoholism. There is a general murmur of approval about not funding this sort of thing (as my mind wanders to Mickey Mantle), but the notion is controversial; a humanitarian country should take care of all its citizens, someone says, and there are widespread murmurs of agreement. Nothing said here strikes me as different from American sensibilities.

When McIver asks more pointedly where money should be found to pay for Tdx, the group identifies a range of options. All agree that the drug industry should be reined in ("The drug companies are holding us for ransom," says one woman) and that development costs should be borne by government or new drugs taken over by government, which could produce them more affordably. A number of people think that there should be a separate NHS fund for "high-cost" diseases that can be drawn on for people with expensive illnesses.

The two hours allotted for this meeting are nearly gone. Daphne Austin, who has been sitting quietly at the back of the room, stands to thank the group for its comments. Her interpretation of the discussions is that there is general support for coverage of enzyme replacement therapy (ERT) by the West Midlands Primary Care Trust. Almost everyone agrees. Austin says that she is appreciative of their time and guidance, but she asks that those who believe that ERT should be covered provide some additional advice. She says that if in her report to the trusts she were to recommend coverage of ERT, she also would need to identify services to cut, to afford the new treatment. She wonders what suggestions they had. Should they get rid of the diabetes nurse program, for example? One man says "no" with the vehemence that comes from personal experience. After a moment he adds, "You have a bit of a sticky wicket here to deal with. I don't envy you."

Everyone nods. We all see his point. It is difficult to bear responsibility for allocation decisions such as these. No one present wants to say no to someone with the misfortune of having a devastating but costly disease. A health care system with a lean global budget certainly needs to be efficient, but maximizing the aggregate of health for the least amount of money risks the danger of creating fundamental equity problems. Why, indeed, should the life or health of someone with an expensive disease be valued less than the life or health of someone with a reasonably priced problem? Why should government pay to treat some illnesses and not others, given equal effectiveness (or ineffectiveness) of therapy? These are quandaries shared by Americans and Britons alike. I am thinking about U.S. "basic" health benefit packages that pay only so much and no more per calendar year and insurance that leaves out services such as mental health and dentistry. And about differential access by disease in our own version of universal coverage, Medicare, where failed kidneys gain you immediate coverage no matter what your age, but a failing heart or liver requires a two-year wait until disability, and hence eligibility, kicks in.

Unlike others in the room, I envied Dr. Austin. I envied her because the system she works in has decided to grapple with murky ethical issues in a relatively transparent fashion. At policy levels and increasingly with the lay public, considerations of cost-effectiveness and resource allocation are spoken about plainly.

Making Earnest Efforts

Coverage decisions such as the one the West Midlands was grappling with occur when there is a policy vacuum at the NHS level—specifically, when NICE (the National Institute for Clinical Excellence) hasn't yet ruled on an issue coming before local authorities. NICE is the entity to which the NHS has given authority to make decisions about coverage for new or controversial existing therapies. Reporting directly to the Department of Health, NICE was established in 1999 to help improve quality of care, use evidence to inform treatment, and heed issues of economic efficiency within health care treatment. NICE's influential appraisal committees review reports on the effectiveness and cost-effectiveness of new or common therapies. Consulting with patient representatives, scientific and industry reviewers, and, importantly, a citizens council, the appraisal committees deliver opinions on whether the NHS should provide a particular service. This process has by no means fully evolved. NICE is struggling with how to make best use of its citizens council, which is fashioned to represent the U.K. population and which hears "testimony" from expert "witnesses" before coming to its verdict. There is no specific, endorsed method, locally or nationally, for gathering and incorporating public input into health care decision making. But serious efforts are being made to bring the public in.

Once these committees appraise a therapy favorably, it must be made available, when clinically indicated, throughout the United Kingdom. NICE's authority is meant to denote a political and professional judgment that "post-code rationing" (referring to the U.K. equivalent of U.S. ZIP codes), where health authorities in different localities arrive at different judgments about the services they will provide, is not acceptable public policy.

This is not to imply that post-code rationing is a thing of the past or that the British public has accepted "priority setting" as fine and dandy. What is different in the United Kingdom relative to the United States is the British policy focus on equity and the efforts being made to learn what the public thinks and why. The objectives for these conversations appear to be as much about informing and educating the public about dilemmas as about obtaining the public's advice. For the sake of comparison, the most visible U.S. example of soliciting public opinion on health care coverage, the Oregon Medicaid experiment, used public meetings to discuss health care priorities. Nearly 70 percent of attendees, however, were health care providers, not consumers.

Taking a Page from Britain's Book

The Wolverhampton meeting—and a three-day gathering of NICE's citizens council that I also attended—suggested that the deliberation process creates a rich public understanding of and sympathy for problem solving. Canadian and U.K. investigators have found that people may well be willing to leave some of the sticky-wicket decisions to professionals but that learning what the issues are gives them more ease in doing so. At the same time, such discussions provide insights into what the public will and will not accept, better locating policy directions within the value structure of a community and a nation.

While I was sitting in that room in Wolverhampton, the Medicare Modernization Act of 2003 was being signed into law. Like many others in U.S. policy circles, I was aware of the law's unsatisfactory distribution of dollars. Its putative centerpiece—a much-needed drug benefit for older Americans—had been vastly curtailed. A large part of the law's $600 billion price tag was designed to encourage the growth of private-sector health care provision to the Medicare population. It appeared that special interests had been listened to but that the public—the voice of the payers of this U.S. version of universal health care—was missing. Many months later, much of the American public has become aware of how little that legislation has benefited them. Perhaps the widespread discontent with the law will cause Congress to revisit it. Maybe by the time it does, we will consider following our U.K. colleagues by turning to the public for guidance.

Our health care system has become increasingly committed to "shared" decision making in the clinical setting. At the level of the individual, we have moved to educate and offer choices to patients and consumers about their care. We make ever-greater efforts to ensure that communication strategies are sound and that patients participate knowledgably in decisions that affect not only health status but life and death. We view this, correctly, as contributing to the quality and responsiveness of the larger health care system. Our next great wave of empowerment will come when we begin to think at the population level by asking the public for its views on the health care system: What should our country provide, and how should it be paid for? These are no less life-and-death decisions than those made at the bedside. Listening to public voices could help us move our stalled efforts at health care reform forward in a publicly responsive and responsible way. Maybe we'll even adopt the tradition of afternoon tea. Worse things could happen.

⌒ Doctors Have Patients,
Governors Have Citizens

A former governor speaks out about the culture and value clashes between medicine and public policy.

RICHARD D. LAMM

Despite eight years as a Colorado legislator, I knew very little about health care when I was inaugurated governor in 1975. In those days a state legislator didn't need to understand much about health policy. The legislature funded Medicaid, but the program ran mostly according to federal regulations. Health care was growing at more than twice the rate

Volume 19, Number 5: 173–179. September/October 2000.

of the economy, however, and I felt it could no longer be ignored. A governor is reelected or defeated in good measure by how he or she manages the state budget: Basic self-interest demanded that my administration explore this explosive rise in health costs and identify the options available to expand health coverage to the medically indigent. Today, thirteen years after leaving the governor's mansion in Denver, expanding access to the system and controlling health care costs remain my major interests.

In the legislature I had represented a blue-collar district that included union workers, firefighters, shoe clerks, fast-food workers, and small-business owners—hardworking people with big hearts but small budgets. Families in which both parents worked but often could not afford to go to a movie, and those without health insurance coverage through their jobs, generally went uncovered. I had seen, through the political process, what physicians often don't see: men unable to get their hernias repaired, children without access to procedures to fix correctable birth defects, and women without adequate prenatal care. The 600,000 uninsured in Colorado were not mere statistics to people in the neighborhoods I had represented—they were the people I represented. These people didn't want much from me or from government except that we be honest and careful with their tax money—which at the time was scarce for new programs.

I asked our budget people if we could take some existing health spending and use it to provide health care for the working poor. They responded that substantial excess capacity existed in most of Colorado's hospitals and medical practices. This opened my eyes to the great contradiction of health care in this country: In my state, as in most others, surplus capacity in the medical infrastructure consumed large resources, while hundreds of thousands of state residents went without health insurance. In my mind, health care became a metaphor for America: It is filled with good, loving, dedicated people and awesome technology but is awash with redundancy, inefficiency, and unmet needs. It does too much for some and not enough for many.

Working at Cross-Purposes

One area where Colorado avoided excess was in its schools for health professionals. The University of Colorado Health Sciences Center in Denver has been the intellectual epicenter for health care practice and policy in the state. I thought of the center as a necessary ally in expanding health coverage for the state's medically indigent. Turning to the center for a solution, I discovered that like similar institutions, it saw the excess capacity in the system but not within its own walls. Like most other public and private institutions in Colorado, the center had ambitious plans for expansion. Its committed, well-meaning doctors practiced "spare-no-cost" medicine on those lucky enough to be admitted, while nearby were half-empty hospitals, underused medical technology, and more specialists than needed. Physicians focused so much on their specialties that they didn't see the unmet needs around them. They favored universal coverage but were unwilling to give up any of their functions or any of their funding.

Nobody owned up to the problem of the medically indigent: not the Health Sciences Center, the state's practicing physicians, the hospitals, or the professional organizations. When I asked the chancellor of the center why Colorado taxpayers were helping to train so many specialists who often moved out of state when we needed family practice doctors, he pleaded that they were doing desperately needed research. Was that enough of a reason to train surplus medical specialists, when the money could buy more health by covering the medically indigent? The Health Sciences Center was busy pushing up the ceiling of medical possibilities while I was trying to build a floor under those who had no coverage.

Colorado's doctors were constantly reminding me that in medicine "cost was never a consideration." But health care was the fastest-growing segment of my budget, demanding increasing amounts of public funds for the medical school, for new equipment at the hospital, and for Medicaid. Daily, if not hourly, hospitals in my state would effectively appropriate state funds for a high-risk, low-benefit procedure, while I knew that those funds could easily save more lives elsewhere in the health care system or outside of it, say, by buying three new teachers, fixing a broken sewer main, or adding two police officers to a high-crime area for a year. How could cost not be a consideration in making a public budget?

In the tight little universe of patient advocacy and health provider professionalism, health care providers were allocating taxpayer funds and insurance funds without regard to any other uses of the money. Taxpayers now fund about half the costs of U.S. health care (much of it through Medicaid and Medicare, which are "entitlements"), yet the legislative process demands far less accountability for these monies than it would in other areas of government spending.

Two Cultures

Clearly, a wide cultural gap exists between deliverers of health care and tax-payers who increasingly pay for that care. Medicine is a culture of "do no harm," while public policy—my culture as governor—is trained to maximize good. One culture demands all that might benefit a particular patient, while the other builds systems in which you can never do everything of benefit and where it would be foolish to try. How do we reconcile those whose duty it is to micro-allocate medicine with those whose duty it is to macro-allocate public resources? While I was governor, I often asked myself, "How can patient advocates feel so good about the system they work in when I, as public advocate, feel so guilty for having so many people without even basic health care?"

The clash of cultures between the patient advocate and the public advocate was never so clear as when, in the late 1970s, famed liver transplant surgeon Tom Starzl wanted to expand the transplantation program at the University of Colorado Health Sciences Center. When I was governor, Starzl was not only one of Colorado's leading doctors, but he was also a leading citizen and a friend. His dedication to and promotion of transplantation illustrates the different moral universes of medicine and public policy. He wanted more staff, more resources, and more emphasis on transplantation. I felt that Colorado's next priority should be expanding coverage.

Each of us argued our cases publicly between 1976 and 1981—at state budget meetings, in newspapers, and at public events at the Health Sciences Center. Despite our best efforts, however, the dialogue seemed to occur between the blind and the deaf.

In 1987 (see *Dialysis and Transplantation* 16, pp. 432–433) Starzl wrote eloquently about the needs of the individual, citing two patients who had recently greatly benefited from a liver transplant. One was a thirteen-year-old girl with acute liver failure who received a liver transplant (cost: $87,000) and who, seven years later, was living a normal life on the farm on which she was raised. The other was a seventy-six-year-old woman, who subsequently passed the five-year post-transplant mark (cost of transplant: $240,000) and lived a full life at home. Wrote Starzl in comments not published in the journal carrying the debate but later published in his 1992 book, *The Puzzle People: Memoirs of a Transplant Surgeon*, "The transcendent status of human personality is the bedrock of our secular, pluralistic society. The taking or debasing of life by withholding effective treatment ought not to be justifiable *no matter how great the offsetting 'benefit' to the public good"* (emphasis mine).

I wrote about all the other unmet medical needs in Colorado. It was unthinkable for me to expand the transplantation program when 600,000 state residents lacked basic health insurance. It was unthinkable for Starzl to turn down anyone who might benefit from a transplant. When I asked why we had to duplicate transplantation facilities available in other states and suggested that Colorado should cover our medically indigent first, he accused me of being anti-research. I countered that research was wonderful, but I was first in favor of maximizing the health of Colorado. To Starzl, I was backing away from a world-class program. In his words, "The failure of Mr. Lamm to take advantage of what has happened under his own sponsorship [referring to the success of the University of Colorado transplant program] is like giving birth to a beautiful child and then trying to starve it so that it will not threaten the food supply." Neither of us was soft-spoken.

The center of a doctor's moral universe is the patient, and the doctor's role as patient advocate has been an important part of two thousand years of medicine. Starzl was not about to let anyone die if he could avoid it, no matter what the cost, no matter the other health needs of Colorado. Foreshadowing a dialogue that would explode a decade later with the rise of managed care, I felt that money could save more people if it were spent elsewhere in the system. I felt a moral responsibility to maximize the dollars that are so painfully plucked from the pockets of my constituents and to weigh all public needs in deciding which unmet needs to address. Starzl believes that America has the "best health care system in the world," but I disagree. Our system is inadequate because it doesn't permit all Americans access to medical miracles, only those with health insurance coverage or the ability to pay out of pocket for medical services. An educational or highway system would never be considered adequate if it left 14 percent of its citizens without schools or transportation, as was and still is the case for the 14 percent of Colorado residents who lack health insurance.

Saying No to the Doctor

Tom Starzl is a superstar and I honor his accomplishments, but Colorado needs basic health care for its medically indigent before it needs a world-class transplantation program. It is easy for people to ask, "Why not have both?" but making a budget is the deepest expression of one's values and priorities, and I felt that Colorado taxpayers' next priority should be to expand coverage.

"It was a pity to terminate the discussion," wrote Starzl. "Mr. Lamm's was a description and defense of statistical morality, and mine was the same justification of the doctor-patient relationship which I had used as my lifetime ethical standard."

Starzl's final written rejoinder captured perfectly the conflict between medicine and public policy. The health provider's tool kit contains the miracles of modern medicine and pharmacy, but public policy has a wider range of options, including public health, education, smoking cessation, highway safety, and so on. Tom Starzl is a great doctor because he concentrates on his specialty and applies it with great caring to individual patients. But his compassion was trumping other important health needs such as expanded basic coverage, which I felt could have improved health for more people.

The exchange with Starzl, both verbal and in the literature, still haunts me. He is absolutely right, according to his culture. But walk awhile in my shoes. In a world where cost is inherent in every decision, how do public policymakers fund the needs and demands of a profession where "cost is no consideration?" How do we compare health care needs with other important social priorities?

Starzl is not alone, of course. The American public has come to feel entitled to what no nation can financially deliver—all the health care that is or may be beneficial to its health. The dilemma of democracy is that citizens want more services as consumers than they are willing to pay for as taxpayers. The ultimate challenge to an aging, technology-based society is to adjust public expectations and medical practice to what the society can realistically afford.

It will not be easy, but it must be done, for no item of public or private budgets can continue to grow at twice the rate of inflation. Ultimately politics has to adapt itself to reality. Jacques Chirac of France once said, "Politics is not the art of the possible, it is the art of making possible what is necessary."

Seven years after my written exchange with Starzl, a brilliant political leader and a physician, Oregon governor John Kitzhaber, with the support of the state medical society, implemented the Oregon Health Plan. The governor's desire to expand health insurance to more low-income people was driven by firsthand experience as an emergency room physician, where he saw the tragic results of Medicaid cuts.

The Oregon Health Plan was controversial when first proposed in 1989 because it added many uninsured people to the Medicaid rolls by reducing the Medicaid benefit package. The goal was to cover more people but for fewer services. The state created a prioritized list of 700 services and treatments, ranked in order of importance; the Oregon state legislature drew a line at item 587. Treatments below the line—deemed to be less effective—would not be covered. The plan went into effect in early 1994. As of 1997 the plan had added 100,000 people to the Medicaid program. In the words of a physician who evaluated the program, "Serious complaints about the prioritized list are hard to find" (Thomas Bodenheimer, "The Oregon Plan—Lessons for the Nation," *New England Journal of Medicine*, 28 August 1997). Among the treatments not covered by Medicaid in the plan were organ transplants in cases where the need for a transplant was deemed low on a severity scale.

Governor Kitzhaber was able to persuade Oregon legislators and voters that when a state fails to provide health care coverage for all of its medically indigent, it already is rationing health care. "We are like high-level bombing planes whose pilots don't see the faces of the people they kill," he often said. The decision for a state isn't *whether* to ration but *how* to ration. With the support of Oregon's medical and hospital societies, the governor demanded that the state prioritize its Medicaid funds. The real question for our states is not whether a system of priorities like that adopted in Oregon is ethical. The question, instead, is whether it is ethical for a state *not* to have a prioritization system for health care coverage.

The house of health ethics and policy has more than one floor. The first and most important floor is the doctor-patient relationship, but it is not the only floor. Health plans are also fiduciaries of the funds they collect. Likewise, the state is a fiduciary of the funds it collects from taxpayers. When exercising its moral duty as fiduciary, a state cannot be judged by the doctor-patient relationship.

As Sir Francis Bacon said when arguing that the inductive reasoning of the scientific method should not be judged by the deductive reasoning of the Aristotelian system, "I cannot allow myself to be judged by a tribunal that itself is on trial." Neither can the actions of a state or health plan be judged solely from the viewpoint of doctor-patient medical ethics—not when doing so prevents us from serving the broader health care and other needs of the tax-paying public.

∽ *Hooked on Neonatology*

A pediatrician wonders about the hidden cost of NICUs' success.

JOHN D. LANTOS

I almost fainted during my first visit to a neonatal intensive care unit (NICU). I was a fourth-year medical student. The babies got to me. Some of them were pink, others a bit grayish. Some were in diapers and seemed to be looking around. Others were blindfolded and lying naked under banks of fluorescent lights. The basinettes of some were wrapped in cellophane. All were connected to machines and monitors—mechanical ventilators, cardiac monitors, intravenous infusion pumps, intra-arterial pressure gauges, temperature sensors. Shameful to say, the babies evoked in me a strange mixture of sympathy and antipathy. Their vulnerability made me want to care for them, protect them. I wanted to join the devoted staff, whose energy, science, and devotion almost created an artificial womb to keep these tiny marvels alive. But there was also something disconcerting about their dependence on the machinery and medical technology—and about their dependence on us.

A Stranger's Queasiness

Nurses hovered over each basinette. They would occasionally pick up or turn a baby, but mostly, it seemed, they watched the monitors, keeping the buzzers from buzzing and the beepers from beeping. They would periodically measure medications in tiny syringes and inject them not into the ba-

Volume 20, Number 5: 233–240. September/October 2001. Adapted from *The Lazarus Case: Life and Death Issues in Neonatal Intensive Care* (Johns Hopkins University Press, 2001).

bies but into the tubes connected to the babies. At other times they would withdraw tiny amounts of blood. After each glance at a monitor, injection, or blood draw, they would calmly document the events on the graphs and grids of their thick notebooks.

The babies themselves did not seem central, except in a mechanical way, to the dramas being enacted. In that way, though, they were a crucial part of some vastly complex loop, the energy source to which all else was connected. They were clearly the place where the tubes and wires and catheters came together. Oddly, they were not where the eyes of the professionals focused. Instead, the professionals listened to the rhythm of the beeps; they watched the flickering digits on the ventilators and the infusion pumps and the tracings of the electrical activity of the babies' hearts.

The doctors, nurses, and respiratory therapists talked to one another easily. Their language was the mysterious argot of numbers and abbreviations that technicians everywhere use. They'd casually say things like, "This 26-weeker has RDS and a PDA, he's on a rate of 30, PEEP of 5, 35 percent O2. Neuro: an ultrasound yesterday showed a Grade II. Nutrition: he's down 300 grams since birth, we're starting TPN today. Heme: he's had 3 cc's out and we're replacing it. Social: parents haven't been in." Right. Sometimes the attending physician would ask a question or two. Other times, not. We'd shuffle en masse a few steps to the next hub. The medical team didn't talk to the babies or to the parents, who had been asked to leave the unit during rounds. The team talked around and through the babies in a way that made my head spin. I sort of understood what they were talking about. But like a visitor to a foreign country who had studied the language a long time ago, I caught mere snippets that were not enough to piece it all together. I wanted them to slow down, to translate a phrase here and there, to allow me to participate. I began to feel like an intruder, an outsider, an alien. The things that were going on were so unusual, yet everybody seemed determined to pretend that they were normal. I wanted to point this out, but I had no voice. I began to feel a growing desperation.

The reality of the room became distant and indistinct, the voices fuzzier and harder to understand. I could feel my heart pounding and the blood rushing to my face. My palms became sweaty. I silently excused myself from rounds and went to sit on a sofa in the parents' waiting room, hanging my head between my knees like an exhausted athlete.

It was not a good day. I felt like an idiot. I wondered if I could really do this, if I really wanted to be a doctor. I was scared of what I felt and of what

I lacked. I was scared of what I would have to do in the pediatrics residency that I was planning to start.

Over time, I tried to blot out that moment. As a pediatrics resident, I spent many months working competently in the NICU without swooning again. The episode only came back to me ten years later, when, as a practicing general pediatrician and bio-ethicist, I was writing a paper about ethical issues in the NICU, particularly about the way doctors learn to deal with the stress of difficult moral decisions. I suddenly understood that the inadequacy and doubt that I felt at that moment were not shameful signs of weakness. They were, instead, crucial personal responses to the NICU's disturbing realities.

The Economics Behind the Miracle

Over time, neonatal intensive care has confronted, clashed with, and in some ways rearranged our consciousness. By developing ways to save the lives of a whole population of babies who once were thought too small to survive, it has changed the way we think about what babies demand from us as a society and about what we owe to them. Neonatal intensive care has changed the way doctors, hospitals, and academic medical centers conceptualize their activities and missions. Partly because of changing patterns of pediatric illness and hospitalization, neonatal care has become the centerpiece of tertiary care pediatrics. Evidence abounds for its powerful effects on how we think about child health care.

Board certification in neonatology began in the 1970s. By 1999 there were twice as many board-certified neonatologists (almost 3,400) as there were board-certified pediatricians in any other specialty. For many years neonatology has dominated the annual meetings of the Pediatric Academic Societies. Studies of neonatologists' work, of the changing morbidity and mortality rates in NICUs, and of neonatal innovations far outnumber studies of all other aspects of pediatrics combined.

NICUs have become not just the focus of pediatric scholarly work but also the economic lifeblood of academic medical centers. This is because the number of inpatient hospital days accounted for by premature babies has increased dramatically in recent years, while the number of inpatient days for children between the ages of one and fifteen has been falling steadily. Non-NICU pediatric admissions accounted for nearly nine million bed days in 1980, but fewer than six million bed days by 1993. This large drop is attributable largely to improvements in care. More diseases are now preventable, through effective immunization programs, than were twenty years ago. Improved outpatient care of patients with asthma and diabetes and those in need of minor surgery has led to more outpatient care, less inpatient care, and fewer and shorter hospital stays.

Nationally, about 53,000 American babies per year are born with a birthweight of less than three pounds. Overall, at today's survival rates, these babies will account for 2.1 million bed days. Just a decade ago survival rates for such babies were 30–50 percent lower, and they would have accounted for only 1.6 million bed days. Over this relatively short time period, non-NICU bed days dropped by 30 percent, and NICU bed days rose by at least that amount. It is because of this trend toward shorter inpatient stays for most children and longer inpatient stays for premature babies that NICUs have become the economic engine that keeps children's hospitals running. The survival of hospital-based pediatrics as we know it is increasingly dependent on the commitment to the technologies and the personnel that enable the survival of extremely premature babies.

NICUs are economically successful because they are medically successful. Through the process of developing NICUs and the knowledge that we have gained, thousands of babies who otherwise would have died not only survive but survive in excellent health. The challenge of incorporating the phenomenal success of neonatology into our understanding of what babyhood is all about and into our self-understanding of what it means to care for the most vulnerable among us has changed the way pediatricians think about themselves, their specialty, and their mission.

Shifting from Preventive to Intensive Care

Pediatrics was once the quintessentially preventive medical discipline. As an organized political force, pediatricians advocated for a public health model that considered interventions in terms of what was good for all children. The American Academy of Pediatrics was founded in the late 1920s in part to counter the American Medical Association's opposition to government support for universal access to preventive care for children. Comprehensive preventive services delivered through institutional arrangements called "infant welfare stations" led to decreases in infant mortality rates that were every bit as dramatic as those achieved by NICUs.

Unlike today's intensive care services, preventive services don't behave well as profit-making commodities. In order to lead to cost savings, preventive care needs to be provided to vast numbers of people at low cost and often by unskilled personnel. The cost savings it produces accrue across society rather than to particular providers. Returns on investment take time and are difficult to link directly to any specific intervention. A powerful critique of such programs, then as now, is that universal preventive services threaten prevailing economic structures by implicitly undermining the individualistic view of both providers and consumers of health care. The economic infrastructure of our health care delivery system requires atomizing the provision of health care services into quantifiable entities that can be charged and accounted for discretely. In contrast to preventive care, intensive care maps perfectly onto this economic infrastructure.

One response to this interpretation of why our society seems to value intensive care over preventive care is that we are simply doing what works. Proponents of this view argue that preventive care worked well in the 1920s and 1930s, when high infant mortality was caused primarily by inappropriate feeding practices. Immunizations worked best in the 1950s and 1960s, when infectious diseases were the leading killers of children. In more recent decades, however, those interventions are being maximally used. Neonatal intensive care is the logical next step, the only intervention that, in a postindustrial society, can continue to lower infant mortality.

But is neonatal intensive care the best, the only, or the most cost-effective way to lower infant mortality? Data from here and abroad suggest that some combination of comprehensive social support, preventive health care for women, comprehensive prenatal care, and easy access to family planning services may be far more cost-effective than neonatal intensive care. Of course, in evaluating these data, what we "believe" can affect what we "know," and the way in which we study the efficacy of neonatal care can color the results. For instance, if we examine the fate of all infants who are born at a low birthweight, NICUs will clearly come out looking quite effective. Another approach is to look not just at what happens to babies born at a given birthweight but at the rate of low birthweight within a society.

Over the past twenty years, as NICUs have proliferated throughout the industrialized world, rates of preterm labor and low birthweight have been rising, both at home and abroad. In Sweden the low-birthweight rate rose from 5.5 per 1,000 births between 1973 and 1984 to 6.7 per 1,000 in 1988. In the United States the low-birthweight rate was 7.5 percent in 1997, the highest rate since 1974. The rise in these rates, by itself, would lead to an increase in infant mortality unless countered by improvements in neonatal intensive care. Infant mortality rates are dropping in both the United States and Sweden, reflecting a delicate balance between the rising rates of premature birth and the effectiveness of neonatal intensive care in lowering birthweight-specific infant mortality.

But why are low-birthweight rates rising? It almost seems as if society, by some mechanism, is working against health to produce more and more low-birthweight babies, and that medicine is then working against society, desperately trying to patch the wounds caused by some nameless thing that is forcing our babies from the womb too soon.

A Value Choice

Perhaps the thing is not so nameless. Premature birth is clearly associated with a number of social and economic factors, including the availability of health care services. In Scandinavian countries, which boast the lowest infant mortality rates in the world and some of the lowest rates of low birthweight, these factors are considered in decisions about how to best target resources to maintain the low rates. In the United States the effects of social factors are well studied and even more dramatic. But we do not see these effects as being amenable to intervention because we don't use our economic and political creativity to facilitate or reward the development of the kinds of systems that might modify these factors. Instead, the social and economic environment is viewed as an immutable background against which clinicians, scientists, and hospital administrators work their wonders.

But the political and economic arrangements in which we live have as much effect, or more, on the health of children (and adults) as do the particular clinical interventions we undertake. To a certain extent, neonatal intensive care has become necessary because we have created a society that produces a lot of premature babies. And we have responded marvelously to this problem. We have figured out not only how to develop the science, technology, and pharmacology that will allow us to save babies, but also the financial arrangements that will encourage hospitals to do so. This financial commitment is a sort of moral commitment, but in that sense, it is also a value choice. We reward one type of response to the moral demand of infant mortality (neonatal care) and not another (preventive care).

NICUs make money only because they implicitly make a compelling moral claim upon society. This claim insists that we not turn our back on these tiny, vulnerable babies. It constructs the NICUs as the epitome of our humanity, the measure of our devotion, the test of our will. NICUs stand for our society's moral commitment to children, our excellence in caring for them, and even for our moral progress over time in recognizing that our tiniest citizens have rights. In allowing each preemie to make a moral claim upon us, we see ourselves as altruistic and superior to other cultures in other eras that didn't recognize the common moral humanity of the newborn.

We imagine that we are working to protect premature babies because they need us, but it turns out that preemies are also working for us. They perform an important altruistic function for our medical centers. We are supported by the rewards that doctors and hospitals claim for meeting the obligations that we've taken upon ourselves. Pediatrics departments and children's hospitals are now financially dependent on NICU preemies. At the University of Chicago, for example, over the past three years, the NICU has had the highest revenue-to-expense ratio of any unit in the entire hospital, including both adult and pediatric units. Recognizing this fact, the new University of Chicago Children's Hospital, like most new children's hospitals, will have more NICU beds than the current one but will not have room left over for a new emergency department, new outpatient clinics, or an auditorium for public gatherings.

Societal Messages

Economic realities influence choices in subtle ways, making certain solutions to certain problems seem preferable to others. I do not believe that individual neonatologists decide whether to continue or stop treatment for a particular baby by calculating the reimbursement for care that they or their hospital will receive. But I am convinced that the economic "vote of confidence" given to neonatal intensive care is quite different from the economic "vote of no confidence" given to outpatient general pediatrics, mental health care, dental care, and programs to prevent injuries. That societal message then gets translated into a system whereby parents are charged with child neglect or even manslaughter for refusing neonatal care for their marginally viable babies. Doctors are sued for withholding treatments for particular preemies. But society itself is absolved of the much larger neglect that allows one-third of our children to grow up in poverty. Such spectacles reflect and create a moral environment that is both odd and compelling.

Neonatal intensive care is one of the triumphs of modern medicine. Babies who inevitably would have died a few decades ago routinely survive today. But the success of NICUs should not lead us to see them as the only solution to infant mortality or as an adequate moral response to our children's health needs. We should constantly remind ourselves that the need for so much intensive care for so many babies is a sign of political, medical, and moral failure in developing ways to address the problems that sustain an epidemic of prematurity.

Someday, we will understand the physiology of premature labor and come up with ways to prevent it. Without premature babies, NICUs and the moral and political dilemmas they create will be moot. In the meantime, NICUs are necessary to us in many ways. But they shouldn't control us. In devoting so much expertise and so many resources to neonatal intensive care, we should think clearly about the choices we are making and the choices we are thereby rejecting.

⌒ Here Comes Trouble

A nurse practitioner ministers to a mentally retarded patient's needs while questioning the cost to Medicaid.

KAREN ROBERTS

As I prepared to walk into the room, my nurse handed me a chart, saying, "She's not too happy." She meant Margie, a "frequent flyer" in our office, whom I was seeing for the first time. I knew her by sight, of course, having seen her and her husband in the hallway many times. Many people in our community know them by sight.

I walked through the door. Margie, a round woman in her fifties with flame-red hair that today is in two Pippi Longstocking tails, sits in the chair,

Volume 24, Number 1: 240–242. January/February 2005. The names in the story have been changed.

mouth set in a hard line, refusing to make eye contact. She is unhappy that she is not seeing her regular doctor. Her husband, Albert, however, a slim, dignified-looking man and quite a natty dresser, nods pleasantly and says, "Iiii uhn, owa ooh?" This is to be my first lesson in Albert-ese, a language in which, three years later, I am now fluent. After a moment, my mind translates this to, "Hi, hon, how are you?" and I respond warmly. Albert and I visit, and I gradually pick up the cadence of his speech, affected by both tardive dyskinesia and a lack of dentures—he doesn't like them. Margie looks on, the sullen look on her face gradually thawing until she is forced to jump in. Albert has just finished telling me that Margie won't take her medicine because she's stubborn and won't listen.

"Shoot, I listen to everything," Margie says. "He's just being ornery!" Margie begins to talk, becoming more animated as minutes pass. She tells me her stomach hurts, that she feels "no damn good," that she wants to have a baby. I review her chart while, referring to me, she chatters to Albert (Daddy), "Looky, Daddy, how pretty she is and she's wearing my favorite color, too. I bet she's ornery, just like Dani and Susie [two other nurses in the practice]. Are you ornery?" she demands.

"Well . . ." I cast about for an answer. Margie laughs delightedly. "See, Daddy, she knows she's ornery—I bet she's Trouble. You're Trouble, all right, Pumpkin." Despite my protestations, by the end of the visit I am clearly Trouble, and one of Margie's new favorite people.

Margie likely falls into the category of a person with mild-to-moderate mental retardation. Albert has a mostly unknown history. We assume that antipsychotics caused his speech deficits. They are two of the most un-self-conscious people I have ever met. When they are in the office, everyone knows it.

I am to discover that most visits follow this pattern: Margie presents a pitiful countenance, one that gradually brightens as the visit wears on, to the point of absolute radiance by visit's end. Our interaction is clearly therapeutic. Her typical complaint is abdominal pain or respiratory infection. Fortunately, most times nothing serious is wrong. I say "fortunately," because Margie is a patient who rarely complies with treatment. I don't classify her as strictly noncompliant, though, because Margie cannot read. Her ability to follow the treatment plan is limited. When I treat her, I make little charts with pills taped to the paper, showing her how many times a day to take them. Sometimes she brings large bags of medicines that she has not finished. We sort through them, keeping the ones she needs—allergy, laxative, blood pressure pill, "nerve" pill. I destroy hundreds of dollars' worth of medicine.

At the end of each visit we have social time, for which I am prepared. Margie waits for me to comment on a new t-shirt, hair bow, or piece of jewelry that Albert bought for their anniversary. They celebrate by the month— I think they're now up to fifty-six. Albert dotes on her—taking her to dinner, to the casino, dancing. They are very romantic. I give Margie my pen, which she blatantly covets from the moment I enter the room. At the end of the visit Margie will stop to say hello to all of her favorite staff, even if they are in the middle of work. Albert, like all long-suffering husbands, wisely goes to wait in the car. Eventually, after hugs and kisses and loud accusations of orneriness in general, Margie will leave.

I've also discerned a rhythm to the frequency of her visits, a tempo that keeps pace with the intensity of external life events. When Margie is unhappy about something or is having trouble with her neighbor—a frequent point of conflict—I see her more often. Lately she's been coming about once a week. Some days my heart sinks when I see her on my schedule. Despite my affection for her, she is frustrating because essentially there is nothing wrong with her. We worry, however, about missing something, so I work her up, within reason. I rely mostly on a careful history of recent life events to tease out what brings her to my exam room.

Riding the System

One of the reasons I can do so little for Margie is that her problems are mainly psychosocial. I can and do provide social support, but she is convinced that something is physically wrong with her. Her symptoms often escalate if we refuse to see her. She also tends to doctor-hop. She has Medicare, which requires no referral, and she has an open Medicaid card so she can go to whomever she pleases. She has seen most of the other providers in town, sometimes the day before she sees me. If we make her wait too long, she might also go to the ER.

This is a big part of our frustration. Margie's overuse of medical care concerns us. She is a poor historian and signs few releases. Consequently, she is overtreated or given duplicated treatments, and each layer of privacy legislation fragments her care a bit more. Once she received two colonoscopies within the same month.

With patients like Margie on Medicare and "open" Medicaid, a case management or utilization review mechanism does not seem to be in place, at least not prior to visits or procedures. I suppose payment may sometimes be denied at the other end, but *someone* ends up paying—usually the provider. This seems to be a real failing of the system. Margie likes to get multiple opinions, and so she does. Other patients do not enjoy this luxury. Her primary care physician and I get frustrated when recalling the hours spent precertifying and preauthorizing traditional insurance patients for a test, visit, or prescription and comparing this with the unbridled and often unnecessary care used by Margie. As we pick up "chart 3 of 3," we say things like, "I can't believe our tax dollars are paying for this. What a waste." We also fear the "boy who cried wolf" effect—that one day when something is really wrong, she will be ignored by an exasperated provider. So we put her on the schedule, her physician and I taking turns seeing her.

Most days we can accept the reason that Margie really comes here: We matter to her. We are the people she thinks of when having photographs made, like the one of her and Albert that hangs on my bulletin board. We listen to her. She pours out her life's sadness and disappointments in the exam room. For example, Margie is postmenopausal, so I gently explained to her that she wouldn't be able to have a baby. She cried. How we are also matters to Margie, so she asks about my husband, my girls. We chat. Most days I examine her, reassure her, and send her home.

It's no burden to me personally, but in a health care system weighed down with expense, it's difficult to see patients accessing medical services merely to experience caring human contact. Where is the gatekeeper who ensures that their use of health care dollars is warranted and wise? Even if patients like Margie were subject to case management services, its main purpose would be to save dollars, not attend to patients' psychosocial needs. Indeed, this duty falls, not to the insurer, but to budget-stretched community services. However, as is often the case in health care, the systems interlock in a cause-and-effect manner. Where is the system to support Margie and Albert, to give them a caring presence in their lives? If a system were in place to ensure adequate social support and to help them deal with day-to-day concerns, perhaps their medical visits would be reduced. I wish in vain for a solution, one that would fix the problem but not leave the patient feeling abandoned. I don't know what the solution is. For now, costly and impractical as it may be, I am the solution. I lift the two-inch-thick chart from the rack on the door and check the chief complaint. Abdominal pain. I sigh silently, then open the door.

"Hey there, Pumpkin! Look, Daddy, here's old Ornery." I look at Margie's open face. Albert smiles at me from the corner. I enter the sweet warmth of the room.

∽ Shopping for Long-Term Care

A daughter questions market theories after watching her parents make decisions about long-term care.

DEBORAH STONE

Before dementia crept up, Mom was a consummate shopper. She has impeccable taste; she savors clothes, furniture, kitchen gear, plants, and most of all, contemporary art. She used to spend her days keeping in touch with friends, gardening, visiting galleries and museums, and shopping. I doubt there was a day of her life, save a few spent in the hospital, when she didn't shop. I inherited the gene, and shopping is one of the things we most enjoy doing together.

People like my mother should be perfect candidates for the kind of rational decision making about their long-term care that the market approach to health policy suggests. They have the mindset: Know your goal; compare, evaluate, and choose the best option at the lowest cost. Yet when the time came for Mom to shop for long-term care, it held no appeal. She'd lost her husband of sixty years. She was slowly losing her mind too, and she knew it. The mother who'd never before uttered a word to me about being lonely or depressed now told me she was both. I naïvely thought that our shopping bonds would help us through this rough patch, but at the mere mention of options—part-time help, a live-in caregiver, a driver, just going to look at assisted living residences—Mom shut down and cut off the conversation.

Volume 23, Number 4: 191–196. July/August 2004.

The Wise Consumer Myth

According to market theory, consumers monitor quality and prices and choose goods that best meet their needs, preferences, and budgets. Supplier competition for these savvy consumers automatically directs resources to their best use far more efficiently than government regulation. From the Capital Beltway to the Ivory Tower, long-term care policy—like the larger health care landscape—is inspired by market thinking. The answers to every problem (cost, quality, loss of autonomy) are to be found in consumer sovereignty. Call it "consumer choice" of insurance plans, as in Medicare+Choice. Call it "informed consent" or "informed decision making." Call it "consumer-driven care." All of these variations on the consumer-sovereignty theme come down to the same thing: Toss the problems back to the people who need care and their families; let them make the decisions; perhaps give them a little money, a voucher, or a budget to allocate—and poof! Costs suppressed, quality monitored, and freedom regained.

It's fairy-tale magic, this market story with Wise Consumer as its hero, and it revolves around fairy-tale characters. I don't know any real people, especially frail elders, who are motivated or think much like *homo economicus*. When I read the policy literature on long-term care, I have to wonder whether the nation might envision better long-term care policy if all the analysts and politicians spent a little more time listening to their parents and a little less listening to each other.

Both my parents stayed blessedly healthy and fit through their seventies. They kept their considerable marbles, too. Dad had run a manufacturing company with great success, then he "retired" to a career in public service. He read ravenously in politics, economics, science, education, and even health policy. Mom, too, is a person of keen intelligence and quick wit. She is well-organized, well-read, and prodigiously talented. My parents are the ideal, best-we-could-hope-for health care consumers. Dad even relished a good epistolary brawl with Blue Cross. They both completed living wills and health care proxies more than a decade ago. But over the past ten years I have helped my father through four hospital stays and my mother through two. I have accompanied them on numerous doctor visits and helped them think through their choices. Trust me, they never thought or behaved like *homo economicus*.

Each time Mom or Dad was in the hospital, somebody brought them a clipboard with lots of papers to sign on the morning of their discharge. Dad usually scrutinized documents to uncover the hidden traps in bureaucratic language and, more often than not, fired off a few letters of protest to his congressmen. Not so the discharge papers. He'd sign them without so much as a glance, muttering to the discharge planner, "If this is what I have to do to get out of here..." Mom didn't have the same habit of studying legal forms, but like Dad, she understood that she needed to sign to get sprung, and that was all she needed to know to apply her John Hancock.

Protective daughter that I am, I would ask to read the forms ex post signature. They were clearly meant to protect the hospital by documenting that it hadn't put anybody out on the streets without consent. The discharge papers also had a disclosure to the effect that Mom or Dad had been offered home health services to be arranged by the hospital, that such services might be provided by an agency owned by the hospital, and that Mom or Dad acknowledged and accepted any such cozy financial relationship. My parents could not have cared less.

Real Behavior

The gurus of long-term care hope that people like my parents can be trained to make decisions about their care and perhaps even to manage their caregivers. For instance, Robert and Rosalie Kane have suggested in *Health Affairs* (Nov/Dec 01) that because a hospital stay often triggers a change in an elderly person's living and care arrangements, we could help consumers like my parents make decisions that are more in tune with their preferences by "training discharge planners and case managers, and allowing sufficient time—that is, paying for longer [hospital] stays—to grapple with the subtle and complex issues involved." "Hell, no!" I can hear my parents grumble. "Just get me out of here." If my parents are any indication, the hospital stay is hardly a teachable moment.

The first time Mom had surgery for lung cancer, her doctor ordered follow-up home care. She was still groggy from anesthesia when Dad and I got her home. Dad told her that the visiting nurses would be coming later on. "Who asked them to come?" she demanded to know. "I don't need a nurse." If she hadn't been wiped out from major surgery, she never would have accepted home health care, even minimal, no matter how blue in the face some discharge planner might have gotten explaining its benefits to her.

By the second time Mom had lung surgery, Dad had passed away. She was living alone, still in mourning, and she was even less able to manage than she had been five years before. This time I took matters in hand. To supplement the home care time that Medicare would cover, I lined up twenty-four-hour aides from the private-pay side of the Visiting Nurses Association (VNA). I would have done it anyway, but one of the hospital nurses told me that Mom couldn't go home unless she had someone with her around the clock. I knew the nurse's "couldn't" was an empty threat in this era of sicker-and-quicker discharge. But I also knew that she was telling me that full-time care was medically indicated, and I welcomed her exhortation as ammunition against my mother's resistance.

I spent a great deal of time explaining to the VNA's care coordinator that Mom opposed having aides, so we needed people skilled at dealing with elders' resistance. About an hour after I got Mom home from the hospital, the agency's admitting nurse and an aide showed up. We all sat down at the kitchen table, Mom full of energy and elated to be home. The nurse gave Mom a notebook, opened it to a page headed "Patient Rights and Responsibilities," and proceeded to tell her six ways to Sunday that she had a right to refuse services. Mom could ask an aide to leave at any time—it was her house, after all—she didn't have to let anyone in if she didn't want, and she could call a toll-free number at any time to end services. "Please tell me the number again," Mom asked. If I hadn't been there, she would have sent the VNA packing right then.

When the nurse was through, I walked her outside and refrained from strangling her while I asked why she had fairly invited Mom to refuse home health care. "It's the new patient privacy regulations," she explained, mentioning some Health Insurance Portability and Accountability Act (HIPAA) regulations that were about to go into effect. "We have to tell patients their rights." A few hours later Mom asked the aide to leave. The aide came to find me in another room. "What do I do?" she asked. "You stay," I said. "I can't," she replied. "If the patient asks me to leave, I have to leave the house." I was incredulous. I thought that *I* had hired these people, not my mother. The aide allowed, "I *am* supposed to phone the agency before I leave and tell them the patient has asked me to go." My siblings and I managed to get Mom to accept a few hours of home health aides over the next week by telling her that "they're for us, Mom, we need a break." But after a week she put her foot down, phoned the agency, and called it quits.

Finding a Compassionate Solution

This is what passes for "consumer empowerment." All of the regulations that supposedly empower my mother to make her own choices about long-term care in fact incapacitate the VNA and any other Medicare-certified agencies subject to these consumer-protection follies. I sensed that if I wanted people who could persuade Mom to accept help instead of accepting her refusals at face value, I needed to hire private caregivers or work with agencies that are not beholden to Medicare regulations.

I phoned a private geriatric case manager and asked if it was possible to find caregivers who would interpret patients' rights more flexibly than the VNA did. Patrick told me a story. One morning an elderly woman with dementia refused to let her long-time aide in the door. The aide went to her car, sat for fifteen minutes, then knocked again at the door and said cheerily, "Hi, I'm here." "Oh, I'm so glad to see you," the client gushed. My siblings and I hired Patrick. We knew that Mom couldn't live alone any longer, but Patrick wisely said that she had to reach this decision herself. He patiently guided her through scenarios, asking her to imagine "what if" she encountered this or that difficulty. What would she like to have happen? Where would she like to be? Over the course of six weeks, Mom went from adamantly refusing to consider even a few hours of part-time help to begging for a twenty-four-hour live-in caregiver.

Mom's decision making was a profoundly sad kind of consumerism. Shopping in boutiques and anticipating where you'll wear a new outfit, hang a painting, or use a new gadget are pleasures. Planning how you'll get by if you can't walk anymore or remember how to use the microwave is not something anyone wants to think about. You can tell my mother that she's in control, but she's too smart to be fooled by empowerment bunkum. She knows that the point of this exercise is that she is losing her powers.

We eventually hired some part-time caregivers for Mom. She asks me alternately, "Can't I have someone here nights, too?" and impatiently, "How long is this going to go on with these babysitters?" Her ambivalence about help is typical of frail elders and defies the economics assumption that people hold consistent preferences. I suppose that the consumer-sovereignty advocates would say that my mother exemplifies their hopes. After all, she came to the decision herself, counseled by a skilled geriatric case manager. She did so, however, with her back against a wall. Patrick didn't so much clarify Mom's options as force her, albeit gently, to stare her future in the face and admit to needing help. I believe his conversations made her feel cared for, not because he "informed" her about services but because she valued his attention, his time, his visits, and his kindness. Most of all, he took the burden of decision making off of her shoulders. He told her, "You don't need to worry about how you're going to cope. From now on, your children and I will worry about everything." Mom said she was relieved.

To be sure, Patrick made Mom feel her wishes would always be respected. He assured her that no one would force her into anything, even though she would be ceding control over her life to others. He gave her autonomy in small and symbolic ways to compensate for the big and real autonomy she is losing.

Services Unwanted but Not Unneeded

The market model is all wrong for long-term care because it imagines care as a good or a service that people want, like a steak dinner or a massage. "There is a real problem with long-term care," wrote economist Mark Pauly in *Health Affairs* (Nov/Dec 01). "Most of the services are not the medical services that healthy people would want to avoid but, rather, are the 'low-tech' or 'servant' services that anyone would find helpful, whether well or ill." But most elders find the very idea of services humiliating, demeaning, intrusive, and a mark of defeat before they come to find the services helpful. For my parents, and I dare say for most postpubescent humans, care is a "bad." No one wants to need it.

Because economists regard care as a good, they are convinced that people want to consume endless amounts of it. If public policies make long-term care free or relatively cheap, the argument goes, elders will break the bank in their eagerness to get all they can. To control "overutilization," policymakers impose cost sharing, asset spend-downs, and other economic deterrents to seeking care. They cut home care budgets and set per case caps so that providers, too, have incentives to stint on services and terminate them quickly. These policies subtly denigrate care and punish people who ask for it. Pride and shame are already deterrents to appropriate use of care. Policy thinkers ought to worry more about how to persuade people like my parents to accept help and less about how to suppress their demand.

The market model is detrimental too, because it sets up a competitive, almost adversarial, relationship between patients and providers. It is unfashionable these days to advocate the kind of proactive, protective — and, yes, paternalistic—care that we and Patrick are now giving my mother. But caring for my parents has convinced me that this approach to care is more effective, compassionate, and caring than the approach that starts with *caveat emptor*. Patrick's sensitive and therapeutic alliance with my mother has nothing in common with the threatening, isolating disclosure notices and rights recitations we now offer elders in the name of informing them and enhancing their autonomy. True care has to start from a painful truth: Someone who needs care is dependent. Pretending that people who need care have only to push their shopping carts around the aisles of life is a cruel hoax on them and an evasion of our moral responsibilities as family members and citizens. My mom seems to know all this: Now in her last months, she repeatedly tells me, "I hate shopping."

～ On Being a Grantmaker

A foundation head sustains others' work while nourishing his own.

MICHAEL LERNER

O n Halloween 1991 Jenifer Altman knew she was dying. She called me to her house overlooking the Pacific Ocean in the small town where we both lived. She asked me if I would be willing to take responsibility for helping her turn her $12 million estate into a foundation. In that moment Jenifer changed my life.

I was forty-eight when Jenifer died. Born in New York, I had taught political science at Yale and had come to California in 1972 on a sabbatical. In the town where I settled, I met a woman who was directing a school for neurologically handicapped children in Berkeley. She introduced me to a little girl who had been diagnosed as retarded until a nutritional therapist had removed all wheat and dairy from her diet. It turned out she was learning disabled, not retarded. I was astounded that diet could affect consciousness. I

Volume 22, Number 3: 183–188. May/June 2003.

resigned from Yale to start a residential school to explore the role of nutrition in the learning and behavior disorders of children.

One day in 1974, after the residential school was up and running, I looked out across the fields at the edge of our town at an old RCA radio transmitting facility nestled among trees on the cliffs overlooking the Pacific. I imagined turning those buildings into a center where we might work at the interface between individual health and earth's health. With a few friends I was able to lease the site for fifty years. There we created Commonweal, a research institute that focuses on environmental public health, programs for cancer patients, continuing medical education for physicians, and work with at-risk children.

Jenifer Altman had come to Commonweal to participate in our Cancer Help Program, a retreat for cancer patients that I still co-lead today. These retreats offer cancer patients a week of yoga, meditation, massage, vegetarian diet, art therapy, and support groups. I lead evening sessions on making choices in conventional and alternative cancer therapies, dealing with pain and suffering, and facing death and dying.

Jenifer felt that the Cancer Help Program changed her life and asked if she could come work at Commonweal. While working with our staff, she continued her fight for life. She thrived at Commonweal. Her face, pale when I met her, filled with color. She began to laugh, to dance, to live—for two years longer than she or her physicians had expected.

I sat with Jenifer, as she lay in her bed facing the ocean, through the days and nights of her dying. We had attended the same school in New York, although years apart. One early morning, just before the light, I sang her the strangely beautiful school song: "We go forth unafraid / Strong with love and strong with learning / New worlds will be made / Where we set our beacons burning." It felt true to me that Jenifer and I had set our beacons burning together in this small town.

Philanthropy's Craft

Being a grantmaker looks easy from the outside. It is not. When I became president of the Jenifer Altman Foundation, I had been asking for grants for twenty years, first to build the school for at-risk children that I cofounded when I came to California and then to build Commonweal. I knew how to ask for grants, but I knew nothing about making them.

The first grantmaker meeting I attended as president of the Jenifer Altman Foundation was a 1992 Environmental Grantmakers Association meeting near Tucson, Arizona. Before this I had only gone to grantmaker meetings occasionally, as an invited "resource person." Attending in this capacity
typically is an agonizing experience for a nonprofit representative. It is like
being a very hungry man staring at a loaf of bread held just out of reach. You
are only allowed there for a few hours to give a talk; you are surrounded by
unimaginable resources yet are forbidden by etiquette from approaching
anyone about support for your work.

Now, as the president of a small foundation, I had magically been transported inside the sanctum sanctorum, the charmed circle of philanthropy.
Yet I still felt very much an outsider. The scene that first evening, as the grantmakers gathered in loose clusters after dinner under the cool, dark desert sky,
reminded me of the court of Louis XIV, except that these gifted courtiers—
the professional staff of a hundred foundations—were dressed in blue jeans
and Birkenstocks instead of silk and satin. They were invisibly but deeply at-
tuned to the modern kings and queens, dukes and duchesses of the philanthropic world—the presidents and senior staff of the larger foundations, and
the family trustees of any and all foundations. By the end of the conference
I was in a state of psychological shock. Such an enormous amount of wealth
was represented there. The dance around it seemed infinitely complex, so
mannered, so nuanced. I did not think I would ever understand this dance,
and I was even less sure that I wanted to. My deepest impulse was to take a
long shower and get as far away from this gaggle of grantmakers as possible.

But I did not get far. I came first to tolerate the funder meetings, then, to
varying degrees, to like them, and finally to depend on them as an integral
part of my work. I found my home as a grantmaker in the Consultative
Group on Biodiversity (CGBD), in the larger Environmental Grantmakers
Association (EGA), and in Grantmakers In Health (GIH). It was in these
grantmaker affinity groups that I found the wise and experienced men and
women who schooled me in the craft of philanthropy.

Choosing a Niche

Eventually we focused the funding work of the Jenifer Altman Foundation
on the intersection of health and the environment. This resulted from my
exposure at a meeting of the CGBD to the shocking new science on

endocrine-disrupting chemicals. This science is demonstrating that some chemicals may have wide-ranging effects on fetal development at exposure levels far below those of traditional regulatory concern.

My interest in this area was due in part to our Commonweal work with cancer patients and children with learning and behavior disorders. The more I learned about traditional toxicology and the new literature on endocrine-disrupting chemicals, the more concerned I was that environmental contaminants might be contributing to a wide range of chronic illnesses (asthma, birth defects, learning and developmental disabilities, cancers, and so on) that are increasing or are at disturbingly high levels. I deeply felt that we have not put enough research effort into exploring the linkages between environmental contaminants and the epidemic of chronic illness we are experiencing.

Environmental health works at the interface of human, animal, and ecosystem health; as a field of philanthropy, it is quite new. Four years ago I joined with other funders to found the Health and Environmental Funders Network (HEFN) to represent the field. (Philip R. Lee, former assistant secretary of health, is HEFN's chair.) HEFN is a virtual network that works by e-mail and conference calls; it supplements rather than supplants established groups such as Grantmakers In Health and the Environmental Grantmakers Association.

What I learned through grant making is that you have to know your target areas inside and out. You need to know the science, the industries involved, and the legislative and regulatory issues. You need to know the scholarly work in the field and the public perceptions of the issues. You have to learn which of the nonprofits delivers on their grant commitments and how effectively, and the probable cost-benefit ratio of each grant. You have to know the other grantmakers in the field, their strategies, and who you can do business with. Above all, you have to develop a theory of social change that points you toward key leverage points where a grant can make a difference, and you have to be open to modifying your theory as events prove or disprove the sagacity of your previous bets.

There are many ways in which a grantmaker can address environmental health issues. A foundation can support research, policy initiatives, education, or advocacy. In advocacy, some of us have come to believe that seeking to modify corporate behavior in the marketplace is one of the most effective ways to move toward a cleaner and healthier environment. The HEFN funders have supported an array of campaigns to reduce the use of harmful chemicals in the health care, education, computer, construction, agriculture, and military industries, among others.

For example, six years ago a group of funders and nonprofits, including the Jenifer Altman Foundation and Commonweal, started a campaign called Health Care Without Harm. Its aim is to "green" the health care sector by reducing mercury, dioxin, and other toxicants in the medical waste stream. This has been a highly successful collaborative campaign that has closed medical waste incinerators at home and around the world, reduced the use of mercury thermometers and other mercury-containing medical devices, and begun to move the industry away from using PVC plastics in medical devices and other industry materials, since PVC is associated with high environmental and health costs. HEFN funders also helped to launch the Keep Antibiotics Working project, which has played a role in reducing antibiotic use in poultry and other livestock factory farms—a key step in keeping antibiotics effective for human use.

Conceptual Models, Long Attention Spans

To be effective, grantmakers need some sort of conceptual model to communicate different elements of a theory of social change. I like to imagine the market-based campaigns that many HEFN funders have supported as staves in a barrel. Each stave represents a different industrial-sector campaign, such as Health Care Without Harm or Keep Antibiotics Working. At the base of the barrel are the grassroots organizations dealing with toxics in the workplace and the community. At the top of the barrel are campaigns such as our effort to win the first international treaty to phase out twelve of the most toxic man-made chemicals. The bands that hold the staves of the barrel together are the great ethical principles of our campaigns: citizens' right to know what chemicals they are exposed to, and the principle that if the preponderance of evidence shows that a chemical may cause extensive harm if released into the environment, it should be regulated with great prudence.

The barrel metaphor helps guide my work; so do my plans to stick to one subject area for the long haul. It is a commonplace that foundations often have short attention spans; the commonplace often is true. I believe it takes a grantmaker at least three years to become competent in a field such as environmental health and five years to gain some basic mastery of it. I have been in environmental health philanthropy for ten years, but I still have a great deal to learn.

One big problem in philanthropy is that many foundations shift their fields of interest every five years or so. Program officers rarely last longer than that in a field, in any case, because foundation interests shift and because they leave for other jobs. That means that many foundations put aside a subject area just as they begin to achieve some real mastery of it. The short span of philanthropic attention, combined with the profound structural difficulties that foundations have in effectively collaborating with one another, make it easy to understand the skepticism about foundations' competence in allocating resources that one finds among many experienced nonprofit leaders.

Psychological Perils

The sense of disorientation and alienation that I felt acutely at that first grantmaker meeting in Tucson has faded. But I still find philanthropy to be a psychologically perilous profession. Philanthropy puts you in a particularly transparent power-mediated relationship with other people. The field's classic urban legend goes like this: A new program officer is taken to lunch by an experienced foundation colleague. The older man tells the newcomer that as long as he remains in philanthropy he will never again have a bad meal or a true friend. Another proverb says that you should not remain in philanthropy more than ten years and that you should have friends from "before" who will tell you when your unearned power has started to erode your integrity. There is wisdom in these admonitions.

Philanthropy is ultimately about providing resources for others to do good work. Most of the pleasure of philanthropy is therefore vicarious. Of course, a gifted and fortunate few people manage to make philanthropy a creative art form all its own. But even they often miss the satisfaction that comes from hands-on work. Some of my friends find great satisfaction in the opportunity to support gifted grantees. They have adapted to the profession in a humble, positive way. Others thrive in unhealthy ways on the power that philanthropy gives them.

My core survival strategy in philanthropy has been to stay moored in my nonprofit work at Commonweal and at the Smith Farm Center for the Healing Arts, where we offer the Cancer Help Program in Washington, D.C. Since I started the Jenifer Altman Foundation, two other friends also asked me—and I agreed—to direct their family foundations. All three of these foundations collaboratively focus on environmental health. They are managed by a very able executive director based in San Francisco, making it possible for me to devote less than a third of my time to philanthropy. That is about right for me.

I continue to live in the small town where Jenifer Altman found me. The heart of my work remains Commonweal's Cancer Help Program. We recently finished our 112th weeklong retreat. Nine people came from across the country looking for the best way possible to live with and, if necessary, die with cancer. At the end of these weeks, I know I have touched lives. I can't say that for making a grant. Deciding on the best possible use of resources is deeply useful. But it does not reach my soul.

I admit to feeling a deep paradox in being both a grantor and grantee. When someone contributes to Commonweal, they make it possible for us to continue work that touches the soul. When I make a grant to support someone else's soul work, I am facilitating what others make possible for me. One would think that I could reach the point of taking as deep a personal pleasure in making possible others' soul work as I do in engaging in hands-on work myself. But that visceral gratitude, for whatever reason, has eluded me in philanthropy. I am deeply thankful for the opportunity to contribute to environmental health philanthropy. But supporting the work of others feels more like a cherished duty than a source of personal creative joy. The joy, for me, comes from continuing the work we do at Commonweal and Smith Farm that other funders have made possible.

CHAPTER 3

BEARING WITNESS

PATIENTS' STORIES

¡Despierta!   DANIEL J. DERKSEN

Pizza Ship   W. RICHARD BOYTE

Where's David?   JANETTE H. KURIE

Maria   MAHLON JOHNSON

Voices from the Clinic: AIDS Then and Now   ABIGAIL ZUGER

The Yellow Baby   FITZHUGH MULLAN

Blind Faith and Choice   RHIANNON TUDOR EDWARDS

⁓ ¡Despierta!

*A physician's stark encounter with the grim human toll of a
preventable public health problem.*

DANIEL J. DERKSEN

We had just spent a pleasant morning with our three-year-old daughter watching mule deer feed at the edge of a high mountain meadow near Chama, New Mexico. Jesse, a recently retired family friend, had showed us where he'd lived while herding sheep as a youngster in the mountains above Tierra Amarilla. The excursion had been a welcome reprieve from hectic lives—mine as a family physician in Albuquerque; my wife Krista's as an OB/GYN.

We headed for home early in the afternoon to avoid night and July Fourth traffic on the winding two-lane highway between Chama and Española, which is northeast of Santa Fe. We did not leave early enough. Twenty miles before Española, a small pickup truck with two intoxicated teenagers had crossed the center line, slamming into an oncoming station wagon driven by a man with his wife and two young boys inside. No emergency vehicles had arrived. A few people stared helplessly at the mangled vehicles. None of the passengers had been wearing seatbelts.

A Country Jaunt Gone Awry

I pulled off the highway. Krista and I sprinted to the collision while Jesse remained behind with our daughter. Trauma is an inadequate description of the carnage we confronted. Two boys, about seven and eight years old, had been dragged from the station wagon and placed on a blanket. Five or six people looked on, unsure of what to do next. Neither child was breathing, although both still had pulses. I wiped the inside of the mouth of the boy

Volume 19, Number 6: 280–254. November/December 2000.

closest to me with the cuff of my long-sleeve shirt and began mouth-to-mouth resuscitation. He was a beautiful child, hardly a scratch on him, but the sweep of his mouth stained my sleeve with blood.

At the time of this accident seven years ago, the death rate in New Mexico for young motor vehicle occupants was more than twice that of the United States as a whole. New Mexico led the nation in alcohol-related motor vehicle crash fatalities, with 26.7 deaths per 100,000 population versus a national rate of 15.6. Those grim numbers have improved somewhat since the bloody accident I witnessed, as has motor vehicle fatality nationwide over the past century. But progress has been uneven in states such as Mississippi, Wyoming, Montana, and New Mexico, which share a combination of risk factors for high motor vehicle fatality rates: miles of rural roads; high speed limits; low per capita income; and lax enforcement of drinking laws, seatbelt use, and speed limits.

The Battle for Two Boys

It was miserably hot. The boy's pupils were fixed and dilated, but his pulse was strong and his skin color pink. My mind was whirling, due to hyperventilation or to the sun. A state trooper arrived and began directing traffic, towering over the boy and me, shielding us from the sun.

Krista was on her knees examining the other child when an orthopedist ran up to offer assistance. They determined that resuscitation was useless. The boy's neck was swollen and bruised, obviously broken. They turned their attention to the small pickup. Both teen occupants were dead, crushed in the collapsed cab. Two open beer cans remained undisturbed in their dashboard holders. Empty beer cans were scattered throughout the cab. The smell of beer permeated the stifling hot summer air.

The opportunity for intervention had passed. Despite laws, seatbelt use is low in New Mexico, and intoxicated drivers are common. More than two-thirds of New Mexicans killed in motor vehicle accidents are not restrained. As many as a quarter of the state's children travel in cars without wearing seatbelts or using child safety seats. Often because of alcohol, New Mexico's highways are some of the nation's most lethal, especially on weekends. The situation is worse on rural highways and Indian reservations. Adult seatbelt use within the Navajo Nation was only 8 percent in 1988, child safety seat use was zero, and the motor vehicle fatality rate was five times the national average, a high proportion related to alcohol. Those dismal statistics only began to change when, in 1988, the Navajo Nation Tribal Council passed a seatbelt law, created educational programs, studied the effect of alcohol on motor vehicle fatality, and provided child restraints at no cost. By 1995, two years after the carnage I saw, Navajo Nation motor vehicle–related fatalities had decreased by 52 percent from 1988, child restraint usage increased from zero to 45 percent, and adult seatbelt use rose from 8 percent to 78 percent. Positive trends, but not good enough.

Yet liquor stores flourish in our small towns, especially close to Indian reservations. The alcohol industry furiously battles all legislation and efforts to address the problem.

Death on All Fronts

Krista and the orthopedist moved on to the station wagon. The boys' mother was propped in a sitting position, her back against the car's front tire. When Krista touched her shoulder she slumped over, dead. Her swollen, bruised face and the oval hole in the windshield suggested the cause of death.

A few feet from me, someone gently pulled a blanket over the boy with the broken neck. The boys' father appeared. He was a large Hispanic man, dazed from the accident. After glancing at me, he pulled the blanket back. His callused hands cradled his son's face. In a mournful wail, he cried over and over, "¡Despierta, mi hijo!" (Wake up!)

The first ambulance dispatched had blown a tire. When the second finally arrived, I had been giving mouth-to-mouth resuscitation for more than an hour. The surviving boy's pulse remained strong, but he never moved, and his pupils remained fixed and dilated. I learned later that he died within a few hours of arriving at the Rio Arriba County hospital in Española. I felt utterly helpless. My efforts had not been enough to save the child.

The father's voice of despair on that lonely stretch of highway will never leave me. Would the family have survived if they had been wearing seatbelts? Would stricter enforcement of seatbelt laws make a difference? Should there be more traffic checks for drunk drivers on holidays and weekends? Would stronger penalties discourage intoxicated drivers? The answers are probably Yes.

A Bleak Landscape

Rio Arriba County, where the accident occurred, is one of the poorest counties in a state that is one of the poorest in the nation. Residents of the county have the highest heroin addiction rate in the United States. Our governor, Gary Johnson, was interviewed on 60 *Minutes* in the spring of 2000 proposing legalization of heroin, while at the same time he vetoed funding for substance (alcohol and drug) abuse prevention and treatment programs.

Almost yearly it seems that a high-profile legislator in New Mexico is prosecuted for driving while intoxicated, usually about the time of the legislative session, near one of the favorite Santa Fe watering holes. The lawmaker arrested most recently had twice the legal limit of alcohol in his blood.

Earlier this year an up-and-coming professional golfer and local Native American hero was arrested and served time for driving while intoxicated, a story that was reported in *Sports Illustrated*. This was his second conviction. He was embarrassed, promised reform, and assured everyone it would not happen again. His work-release program included eighteen holes of golf a day.

It is time for us to awake from our slumber. A person dies every thirteen minutes in a motor vehicle accident on our nation's highways, and many more are injured. Three of every ten Americans will become involved in an alcohol-related car accident during their lifetimes. The carnage from motor vehicle deaths and injuries is a public health problem whose cure requires a change of lifestyle, more effective intervention and education, tougher drinking-and-driving laws, and stricter law enforcement. Prevention and treatment programs, especially in rural areas, are not available or are not covered by health insurance. The paltry number of slots within inpatient and day treatment programs for substance abuse are not meeting demand, and payment by third-party payers for these services is rare.

What Can Be Done?

A man's agonizing loss of his wife and two children and the deaths of the drunk teenagers who triggered the tragedy might have been prevented. To keep the two intoxicated youths off the roads, we might have had more sobriety checkpoints; we could have lowered the legal blood alcohol limit from 0.1 to 0.08 grams/deciliter and introduced zero tolerance for offenders under twenty-one years old. We might have promptly suspended the driver's licenses of the drunk drivers, had they been stopped before the accident. We might have better enforced seatbelt laws, especially those targeting children.

Espousing a more sweeping view of behavior-related prevention, we might enact laws requiring that physicians more consistently perform screening tests for substance abuse during physical examinations, thus better connecting primary medical care with behavioral health. For example, health plans already use some nationally accepted performance benchmarks to measure a range of health care indicators such as immunization and cancer screening rates. If we want to reduce vehicle-related deaths, it is critical to develop metrics similar to the Health Plan Employer Data and Information Set (HEDIS). This data set was initially formed by a consortium of health plans, large purchasers, and consultants to measure the quality of employer-sponsored medical benefits. The consortium then gave the data set to the National Committee for Quality Assurance (NCQA) for further development and implementation. The NCQA now has 250 organizations (representing 400 health plans) that submit annual HEDIS data. Similar standards should be developed for substance abuse screening and for seatbelt and child seat use among publicly funded patient populations. More broadly, requiring states to meet certain outcome measures based on seatbelt use, alcohol-related fatalities, and access to prevention and treatment programs might encourage enforcement of strategies that are already considered effective.

There is reason for optimism. Seatbelt use in the nation jumped from 11 percent in 1981 to 68 percent in 1997 because of better enforcement of seatbelt, child restraint, speed limit, and driving-while-intoxicated laws; improved road construction; safer vehicles; and education programs. But these steps must be applied in a more rigorous, more ubiquitous, and more collective manner—across our state and across the whole country.

For a tormented father on the side of a New Mexico road, policies that *might have* been put in place are not good enough. Despite dramatic improvement over the years, motor vehicle–related deaths remain the leading cause of injury-related deaths in the United States. How many more fathers will have to watch their children die on the road before something is done?

"*¡Despierta!*"

∿ Pizza Ship

Language counts.

W. Richard Boyte

B rian stared intently with gentle but rarely blinking eyes at the two women at his bedside. A blank expression kept his thoughts, if there were any, from the rest of the world. He lay motionless in the large bed. His emaciated limbs appeared painfully positioned by the relentless pull of his uncontrolled and knotted muscles. His thin chest rose and fell with air delivered through a plastic tube. Elastic tape holding the endotracheal tube in place covered most of the bottom half of his face. When the needle pierced his skin, he attempted to cry out. Sound, however, was blocked at its very formation by the plastic tube. In the jargon of his medical caregivers, Brian's condition was summed up as "ND with P," neurological devastation with pneumonia.

Bright red blood filled a syringe, and the needle was removed with a quick jerk. The nurse handed the syringe to a waiting lab technician for delivery. Numbers derived from its contents would determine if Brian could be released from the machine that slowly but rhythmically delivered air to his lungs. The other stranger at Brian's bedside, his physician, had ordered the blood work for this ten-year-old patient with cerebral palsy. Brian had been admitted from the emergency room very early that morning.

"Doesn't he have parents?" the doctor asked as she stood, arms folded, impatiently awaiting the results of the blood work.

"They went to get breakfast," the nurse explained in a hushed voice. She was concerned that the mention of his parents would upset Brian.

"Well, they should be here," the doctor replied. "Happens all the time. They want us to do everything for these pretzel kids and then just run off for a vacation from responsibilities. Wish I had that luxury. Looks like they never

Volume 23, Number 5: 240–241. September/October 2004. The narrative is a short story and its characters are fictional.

even feed him. He'd be better off if they would just choose to let him die next time."

"Please," the nurse said, holding a cautionary index finger to her lips. "He's awake."

"What, him?" the doctor exclaimed loudly. Her face became hardened with indignation. "This POS can't understand anything," she said with the conviction of a seasoned professional.

"He might," the nurse replied meekly.

"No way. All you have to do is look at him to know that."

"What's POS?"

"Piece of shit, of course. You didn't know that?"

With a slight shrug of her shoulders, the nurse fell completely quiet. Both turned their attention to the returning lab technician. In his hand he held the long-anticipated slip of paper. The physician studied the results briefly before ordering the tube removed with a quick confident nod. She was very pleased to know that this badly needed critical care hospital bed would soon be available again.

The endotracheal tube was removed without incident, a simple act for a trained team of medical caregivers. Brian coughed up thick secretions during the procedure. He then returned to his previous state, motionless and wordless. The doctor, duty done, moved on to other tasks.

The nurse looked up from her charting a few minutes later to see that Brian's mother had slipped into the room unnoticed. Brian's face lit up with recognition. He smiled broadly at her before using a very nasal tone to form slowly spoken words.

"Mooommmy. Baaaby gooo hooomme?"

His mother sat on the bed running her fingers through her son's hair. "Yes, baby," she said lovingly. "We'll go home soon." When his nurse stepped up to the bedside, Brian moaned out the word "preeeetttty." She introduced herself again to Brian's mother, who laughingly explained that Brian always said what was on his mind. "Well, you certainly are a sweet boy," the flattered nurse said to him in a singsong voice that made him smile again.

Brian's face lit up in recognition as his doctor returned to the room. The warm broad grin remained spread across his thin face. The doctor did not notice as she approached his mother. She was eager to obtain the information that would verify her suspicion of neglect. After all, a report to Child Protective Services might be in order. Before she could speak, however, she was startled by Brian's excitedly shouted words, "Pizza ship, piiizzaa shiiip."

Brian's mother, confusion clearly registered on her face, turned toward the doctor. "Pizza ship? Brian is a regular parrot, you know. Did someone mention pizza around him?"

The doctor's face burned crimson. Without a word she turned around and quickly exited the room.

⌒ *Where's David?*

Saving neglected and abused children is possible when health care providers initiate a few simple steps.

JANETTE H. KURIE

We found David in a pile. Not the kind you might usually think of—a pile of neighborhood kids having fun, tumbling over each other. We spotted him in a pile of "no-show charts," the daily stack of records for children who don't make it in for their scheduled doctor's appointment.

At the time (nine years ago), our family practice had what we thought was an adequate system to follow up with these children: Letters were sent to the parents asking them to call and reschedule the missed visit. We then filed the chart, expecting the parent to follow through. However, after receiving no response from some parents, we began to wonder if our system might have holes, if some children were falling through the cracks.

Seeing David

I am a psychotherapist who for nine years has been the faculty behavioralist for the Pennsylvania State University/Good Samaritan Hospital Family and

Volume 22, Number 1: 199–203. January/February 2003.

Community Medicine Residency Program in Lebanon, a city near Harrisburg. I teach interviewing and counseling skills to resident physicians and help them identify and work with patients' psychosocial issues such as depression, anxiety, domestic violence, addictions, and parenting concerns.

One October day in 1993, family physician Carol Baase and I started sorting through a stack of charts, looking for clues in progress notes, growth charts, immunization records, and emergency room visits that might tell us who the no-show children were and why we weren't seeing them.

What first caught our eyes about David's chart was the number of missed appointments for this eighteen-month-old (David is not his real name). No cancellations, just a lot of no-shows since his last well-child visit at six months. More disturbing was his growth chart. Instead of curving upward to indicate a height and weight increase, David's growth line swerved south.

We called his mother. She said, a little defensively, that David was just fine. We worked the education points—talked about the need to check his weight, to see how he's doing developmentally, to get him immunized. She agreed to come in. But on the day of his appointment, she didn't.

We called again. We offered more education about the value of well-child appointments, this time in a slightly firmer tone. "OK, OK, I'll bring him in." Again, she didn't. The next time we called, we spoke more forcefully: "Mrs. B., if you do not bring David in for his doctor's appointment, we will be required to call protective services for medical neglect." It ended up taking protective services to physically bring David in.

The nurse who undressed and weighed David left the room in tears. A beautiful, blond-haired boy lay silently on the exam table. Weighing only as much as an average six-month-old baby, he appeared ready to accept whatever fate befell him. We could have given him all of his missed immunizations in one fell swoop and he wouldn't have shed a tear. It takes energy to cry, and he didn't have that. We hospitalized David that day for failure to thrive, a diagnosis of severe malnutrition that is usually the result of parental abuse or neglect, not primary nutritional problems.

David is a prime example of the estimated one million children who are abused or neglected in the United States each year. In 1997 alone 1,000 children died from abuse and neglect; nearly three-quarters were under age four. When you calculate associated spending on health care, mental health, welfare, and crime, child abuse costs more than $94 billion a year. Although states have immunization requirements for children entering school, no law requires that a child be seen for a well-child exam. No regulation can make David's parents bring him into our office.

Rescuing a Child

In our small community hospital, word of the little child on pediatrics spread quickly. At an age when most toddlers are running and babbling and curious about all that life presents to them, David lay quietly in a crib. With paper-thin skin, dark sunken eyes, and the protruding belly typical of kwashiorkor (a syndrome characterized by severe protein and caloric deficiency), David was unable even to sit without support. Hearing rumors of the child, a hospital administrator made a trip to see him. "My God," he asked, emerging from David's room, "where did we ever find that baby?"

"From family practice," answered a nurse. She should have said, "From a pile of no-show charts."

After a few days of added calories, David started responding. Within ten days he gained two pounds. The vacant look we observed on admission began to focus; the blue veins under his thin skin began to fade. Then one day the close attention he had received from the nurses and family physicians paid off. "He smiled," the nurses said. And word of this small step in communication made everyone smile.

At the team meeting with the family to discuss foster care, nursing called hospital security to stand watch. We had concerns that the parents, sensing that David would not be going home with them, might try to grab him and run.

We held the meeting in the children's playroom. David's dad, dressed in a "Born to Raise Hell" T-shirt, took a seat just outside the circle of chairs. A trucker who hauled freight cross-country, Mr. B. never said a word. He slumped in a chair, legs outstretched, arms crossed. I wondered whether the disdain he portrayed was for us or his wife and where those pent-up feelings might go after the meeting. His anger needed to be diffused, but he would not be engaged. I searched his face for what might have been happening at home. Why had he not called for help earlier when he saw David's health deteriorate? Was it fear? Ignorance? Did he and his wife argue about getting help for David? Or did they simply not care about their son?

"Nobody Ever Came to Save Me"

The case for medical neglect began to build. The inpatient team detailed the medical history. A nurse read notes from David's ten-day hospital stay, and a protective services worker reviewed the home visit. David's mother responded defensively to each detail.

A few days before this meeting, during feeding time, I had observed David's mother screaming at him for dropping a piece of peanut butter and jelly sandwich. The nurse tried to educate the mother. "It's really OK, Mrs. B.," she said, gently. "All children this age drop food. That's why we have a linoleum floor, to make it easy to clean up. When he gets a little stronger and his hand coordination is better, he won't be dropping his food as often." David's mom just glared at her. After the feeding, I handed David to her and asked her to change his outfit, damp from spilled apple juice. Mrs. B. held him straight out at arms' length. "What do you want me to do with this child?" she yelled. It was becoming apparent that shouting was her normal tone. Any other child would have cried. David was used to it.

Through the playroom window, I could see security pacing, waiting for the decision. Finally it came. The director of protective services made the call. "Mr. and Mrs. B., I'm afraid we have no other choice, for David's sake, than to place him somewhere for a while where he'll be safe and get the attention he so badly needs." We sat and waited in what seemed like a loud silence.

Mrs. B's eyes were red and welling up with tears. The director continued, slowly and clearly presenting the mandated actions that would be necessary to get their son back home: weekly mental health counseling, parenting classes, developmental services for David, and supervised visitation rights. A resident physician, letting David's mother know that it was all right to cry, passed the tissues.

"You're going to take my child away from me?" she asked. (The father's eyes never left a patch on the floor.) "Where were any of you when I was a child? Where were all of you when my mother locked me in closets? Or when I was starved?" Now the tears, like tiny balls of silver mercury, rolled slowly down her cheeks.

David's mother pointed to a closet. "She kept me in there for days. In the dark. No one ever came. None of you people ever came to save *me*." Then she raised the sleeve of her shirt. "See these burns?" The circle of participants leaned forward. Patches of muted pink skin ran irregularly down her arm. "My own mother did that! I've been a good mother to David. He doesn't have one mark on him!"

David was placed with a foster family for almost a year. A history of the father revealed severe abuse as a child and incarceration as an adult. The parents complied, reluctantly, with the treatment plan, and David eventually returned home.

Now ten years old, David has *petit mal* seizures, severe attention deficit/hyperactivity disorder, speech delay, and hearing loss. He is in special classes for children with learning disabilities. The parents divorced, and the mother has remarried. David, his mother, and his sisters continue to be seen at our office.

Bringing Invisible Children to Light

To us, David was a gift. His small life taught us that we health care providers need to be concerned not only with the children we see before us, but even more with those we do not. How do we reach the "missing" children to learn if they are in danger or if their parents need our help?

Without doubt, some are not being seen because they lack insurance coverage. I am hopeful that universal health care will be forthcoming and provide the assistance these children so desperately need for a decent start in life. But getting children the health care they need involves more than providing financial access. Family dynamics, work schedules, transportation, and cultural and religious beliefs also come into play. In Pennsylvania, for example, the Childhood Immunization Insurance Act mandates that insurance companies cover all childhood vaccinations and immunization booster shots. Yet many insured children remain unprotected.

If universal health coverage won't solve the problem, what about other options? A few states have tried, with mixed results, to improve children's health care by imposing financial penalties on welfare recipients who do not get their children vaccinated. A demonstration project in Maryland in 1992 fined welfare recipients $25 a month for failing to verify that their preschoolers had received preventive health care services. The project failed to increase vaccination rates. A similar experiment in Georgia threatened loss of welfare benefits for families who did not provide proof of up-to-date immunizations for children under age six. That effort produced some positive outcomes, but the ethics of placing financial penalties on already economically stressed families has prompted questions about such programs.

What about mandating care? Legally requiring that children have check-ups six times in the first year of life; again at fifteen and eighteen months; then at two, three, and four years of age (per American Academy of Pediatrics recommendations) may be unrealistic. Also, mandated care is not needed for all children who fail to show up for health care visits, and it is fraught with ethical, legal, and economic problems, not to mention the logistics of enforcement.

Simpler Solutions

In light of the problems with these options, maybe the best course of action is the simple steps we instituted nine years ago with David. Those initial phone calls eventually developed into a family support program, which evolved as the pediatric at-risk population grew. To date, we have identified, tracked, and intervened for some 1,400 children from birth to age six.

After finding David in the no-show pile, we began looking very closely at who else was not coming in. Daily we reviewed the charts of every child who failed to show. We learned that frequent no-shows often are major identifiers of a child or family needing attention. Specifically, we have defined cause for follow-up as two well-child no-shows in the first six months and two or more consecutive well-child no-shows at any age under six.

Our family support program now includes a team of two nurses and a social worker who are funded by the Good Samaritan Hospital as part of its community outreach. They make home visits, conduct parenting classes, consult with schools, address patients' concerns in the office and by phone, periodically review charts, and help our resident physicians in making referrals to community agencies.

The daily review of no-show charts, still at the heart of the program, is probably the most easily replicable action for other primary care practices, not all of which may have the resources we have been lucky enough to procure. However, any office should be able to have someone review the charts of no-show children and look for possible red flags. Health care providers can then follow up with a call or letter, or a request that protective services bring the child in if parents do not respond, as in David's case. What we need to realize is that once a chart is filed back into the system, the child is out of sight, out of mind, and possibly at risk of a real tragedy—like those the public so often reads about in newspapers.

The intervention model that began as a simple follow-up call to David's family is now being replicated at two public health centers in Philadelphia. Maybe there is hope for some of the other Davids in the world when providers can find the wherewithal to make that first phone call to find out: Where is David?

∼ *Maria*

An unexpected meeting between a doctor and a girl with AIDS bears fruit for HIV prevention efforts.

Mahlon Johnson

I was elated to be going home, to be leaving the National Institutes of Health with minimal damage. I had started making desperate pilgrimages here after receiving a scalpel wound while conducting an AIDS autopsy many years earlier. I'd come in search of a miracle that might reverse the moment when a slipped knife turned me, a young pathologist, into an HIV patient. So far, the new therapies had worked. I'd returned to my hurried life and almost forgotten about the virus. But every year I don a patient's gown and return to Bethesda, Maryland, from my home in Tennessee for special blood tests that are the crystal ball to my future.

The NIH researchers had wanted to biopsy a lymph node in one of my legs, if their surgeons could find an enlarged one to cut on. On this trip (my sixth), to my relief, they could not, and the legs that had carried me through thirty years of daily workouts had been granted another reprieve. So after being drained of blood, I was released with no incisions, no stitches, only a

Volume 22, Number 4: 179–183. July/August 2003.

Band-Aid to hide the latest invasion of my flesh. I was free to go home and diagnose disease, not live it.

Usually the NIH's airport shuttle waiting area is packed with patients, many bald or wearing turbaned bandages and dragging black nylon travel bags on wheels. Lost in the vortex of disease, they come hoping that Oz can help them get home, back to Kansas, to something resembling a normal life. For now, the waiting area was empty. I took a seat in the back corner. While checking the shuttle schedule, I heard a voice say, "I didn't hit you."

A young Latina girl and a heavyset Anglo woman in a tan raincoat had just entered the waiting area. They sat down in the row of empty chairs in front of me. The girl, maybe ten or eleven, had brown pigtails sticking out like bent antennae; she clung to a stuffed brown bear with a shiny, worn "V" nose. She looked away, tightened her Walkman's earphones, and pulled the bear closer, flattening his nose against her chest. The woman, hands cupped in her lap, added, "I just bumped you. I didn't hurt you. Why do you say such things?"

The girl turned farther away from her. She watched people leave the hospital lobby and seemed desperate to escape the woman, desperate to enter some other world. She pulled up the frayed wool collar of her old navy jacket, then shifted the bear, as if suddenly aware that he couldn't breathe. She pulled her legs up and curled around her companion, glancing wistfully at the empty space in the corner. Despite these efforts at distance, she seemed strangely tied to the white woman.

"Are you feeling OK?" No response. "Want a Coke?" The woman sounded disheartened. The girl didn't seem to hear. The woman quietly studied the girl, then cautiously reached over to her. When the girl didn't flinch, the woman began to stroke her wiry hair. After a few minutes she stopped, dropped her hands back to her lap, and stared at them.

From Oz to the Airport

On the shuttle van I settled into the back seat. The girl, followed by the woman, slid on to the seat in front of me. In the afternoon light the youngster's face looked older than her thin, childlike frame had suggested. The woman leaned forward and questioned the driver about their drop-off at Baltimore-Washington International Airport. Seemingly reassured, she sat back and looked around the van, smiling faintly when she saw me. I smiled back. "You come up here often?" I asked. She shook her head. "This is our first trip, but, God willing, we'll be back."

"Leukemia?" I asked quietly, hoping it was nothing worse. The mother flinched but didn't respond. She moved her bag to her right side to give the girl more room. I wondered about her reticence. After all, most childhood leukemias could be treated, if not cured. But the girl's demeanor was not that of a hopeful child visiting Oz for a cure. It was that of a wearied conscript who had battled too long. "Acute leukemia?" I whispered again, hoping the query would not penetrate the girl's earphones. The woman shook her head again, her face now contorted with pain. She searched my eyes for signs of trust, then after some hesitation, whispered, "HIV." I nodded slowly, my fears confirmed. "You came to the right place," I told her. "I hope so," she replied. "It's her last chance."

The woman explained that she and her husband, a Miami minister, loved children and had adopted five over the years. Four had been healthy boys, but their last, a newborn girl, had been different. She hadn't gained weight like her brothers had, and by age three she was sickly. Eventually, she got a bad cold that became pneumonia. The doctors said it was *pneumocystis carinii* pneumonia. That's when they discovered the HIV. They sought out the girl's birth mother, but she already had died of the AIDS that she had transmitted to her daughter. The doctors had tested the adoptive mother, the minister, and the boys for HIV—all were fine.

AIDS doctors started the girl on AZT, which for years worked well. But three years ago it failed, and her CD4 (also called t-helper) cells, which organize our defense against infections, started a relentless decline that went unchecked by prayers or newer drugs. They'd tried protease inhibitors. But nausea and diarrhea from the drugs had stripped Maria (not her real name) of twenty pounds. Meanwhile, her CD4 cell count had dropped to 90, well below the waterline for AIDS. As a last resort, Maria and her adoptive mother had come to the NIH's National Institute of Allergy and Infectious Diseases to enroll in a pediatric clinical trial, hoping that new drugs and an immune enhancer might break what was now a free fall. I looked over at Maria, trying to imagine what it would be like to grow up in clinic waiting rooms. I wondered what kind of life she dreamed of having.

Resting her chin on the bear's head, Maria continued to stare from the world of her headphones out the side window. She wrapped both arms tightly around the bear, who was standing stoically on her bluejean-clad legs. We sped along the Maryland interstate in silence, as the mother, deep in thought, gazed out at a marsh lined with cattails making their last stand against the highway. Eventually she turned to me. "The doctors say it'll be several weeks before they can tell if the drugs are working. Even then, they may not work for long." I tried to reassure her about the effectiveness of the new drugs, quietly praying that they would continue their miracles on me, too. But I knew that they hadn't helped some others, and I tried to imagine watching my own child fail to respond to miracle drugs when other people were rising like Lazarus from AIDS's massive tomb.

Tired of Being Sick

Are you an AIDS researcher? she asked. "Not on this trip," I replied. I told her that I had cut myself on an AIDS autopsy. "Oh, no!" she cried, searching my eyes for signs of fear. After a mute moment she shook her head, then looked at me with newfound trust and blurted out, "Things are going to be tough when we get home. It's been easy in the hospital. Maria listens to the doctors. I think she's intimidated by their white coats. But at home . . . she'll go out with her friends, get diarrhea, and stop taking everything for days."

Maria started fidgeting with the dial on her Walkman and glanced at us with a frown. She knew her mother was talking about her. The woman reached over and gently pulled at her headphones. "Maria, this man's a doctor. He has HIV, too! Talk to him." Maria glared at her, the betrayer of her secret, avoiding my sheepish smile. She turned back to the window but then glanced back suspiciously at me as if I'd claimed to be a long-lost cousin.

"You hanging in there?" I asked, trying to sound cheerful. She didn't turn, but shrugged slightly. "A lot of better drugs should be coming out in the next couple of years." I paused to see if she was listening. "They're supposed to work better—fewer side effects. Things could get better if you can just hang on."

Maria turned her head a little and pulled on the bear. The sun reflected off her pigtails and expressionless face. Her eyes held a hint of disbelief, as if still trying to fathom a doctor having HIV. She searched my face for illness. She loosened her hold on the bear but said nothing. Then she whispered, "The pills make me sick!" with an anger and finality that made me wonder if she'd ever take them again. "Me, too," I responded. "But you'll get a whole lot sicker if you don't take them." She pulled up the collar on her jacket, convinced that no one understood her and her private mourning over the loss of her dream for a normal life. "I'm tired of being sick," she said, then turned back to the window and adjusted her earphones.

"Maria's afraid that some kids at her school are starting to ask questions about why she's sick a lot. She's so afraid that someone will see her taking all those pills and spread it over the school and tell Tommy, the little boy she eats lunch with every day. She's sure her friends will leave her." The woman paused and took a deep, tense breath, wrestling with the notion. "But the principal doesn't think so. He thinks it would be better for her to tell the school, not hide it. They're having an AIDS education program." Maria, still fixed to the window, shook her head violently. "She won't even consider it. She won't listen, not even to my husband." Maria pulled up the bear and closed her eyes. Seeing the signs to the airport, the woman grew silent, nervously sorting through her purse as if bracing for their return to a harsher world.

A Heartbreaker

As we climbed off the van, I waited for Maria, seeking one last chance to make her understand the importance of taking the new medications, hoping that she would respond to them and join the rest of us who had. Maria slowly stepped down from the van and moved up the sidewalk away from us, bear under one arm. She searched the sidewalk as if looking for a trap door to escape from her adopted mother, from HIV, and from me.

"How long will it take for you to get home?" I tried again to sound cheerful. She shrugged, barely looking up. "I bet it'll be fun to see all your friends. Your mom says you've got a nice boyfriend." She fought back a smile and looked away. Hopeful that she might be listening, I pressed ahead. "I bet you'll be a real heartbreaker in a couple years." Still looking down, she smiled and started pivoting back and forth. "I heard you might help with an AIDS awareness program at school." She kept rocking. "You can keep your friends from getting sick by talking in school. They won't listen to teachers, but they would to you." She stopped pivoting.

A moment later her mother, towing a big suitcase, came to say goodbye. We exchanged addresses like expatriates in a disquieting land. Then I hugged her and extended my hand to Maria. She took it shyly. I watched as they hurried off, disappearing into the terminal crowd.

Maria Stands Up

A month later I found a worn manila envelope bulging from my mailbox. It was postmarked Miami. Tearing it open, I pulled out a soft blue Bible and a note. They were from Maria's adopted mother.

"Dear Dr. Johnson, I wish you could have been at Maria's school last Wednesday for the AIDS program. We were so proud. It took some coaching but she stood up in front of the whole school and told them about her HIV and that her mother had probably gotten it from a man and then died from it. She stood up there all alone and almost started crying but she was very brave. She told them she didn't want anyone to be afraid of her because you only get AIDS from sex and drugs and she didn't want anyone else to get AIDS and have to take all the pills. The principal was proud too and spoke about how you get AIDS, but Maria was better. After she was done, some of the kids clapped and her friends came up, even her boyfriend. Her best friend even hugged her . . . I thank God."

The Centers for Disease Control and Prevention would tell you that AIDS is expanding rapidly in the Hispanic community, particularly among young women. Recent studies evaluating beliefs about HIV transmission in Hispanic adolescents suggest that compared with teenagers as a whole, this group is least likely to be knowledgeable about HIV transmission or to practice safe sex. Research also indicates that peer education is more effective than the traditional adult-as-teacher model in reaching adolescents, because teenagers are more likely to listen to their contemporaries than to adults. Educational programs led by the heroic Marias of the world who determinedly battle HIV with pills every day could represent the miracle we seek in the struggle to limit HIV infections among the next generation.

We may never know the full impact of Maria's timid speech to her school. But word of her courage, which spread swiftly throughout the Hispanic community, has surely made an impression on a key audience. Undoubtedly, knowledge of her story has saved others. It has inspired at least one rider of the NIH shuttle in his own struggle against HIV.

∽ Voices from the Clinic

AIDS Then and Now

A physician ruminates on the new longevity of her AIDS patients.

ABIGAIL ZUGER

My old patient Nancy phoned me last week. She just wanted to say hello, tell me the good news about her latest blood tests, and see what I thought about a stomachache she's been having.

If anyone had told me a dozen years ago that at the dawn of the new millennium I would still be getting phone calls from Nancy, I would have laughed. It would have seemed impossible for our relationship to last this long.

Nancy and I first met in a tiny Bronx clinic in 1988, in the very dark days of AIDS. The blood test for HIV had been available for about three years; the first antiretroviral drug, AZT, was just out. Most of the patients in our waiting room had been diagnosed with AIDS after a catastrophic infection of some sort and lived for only a year or two longer. Implicit in one's first handshake with a new patient was the understanding that the doctor/patient relationship was going to be very intense—and very brief.

Nancy was one of the first identified cases of the heterosexual transmission of HIV in the Bronx. She could date her infection to 1984; by the time we met, she had survived for four full years and assumed that her time was running out. Other than the nightmare of her husband's short illness and death, she didn't know much about AIDS, but she did know that her husband's doctor, my boss, Jerry Friedland, was the only doctor she wanted at her bedside when she died. When she discovered that he had lightened his patient load and bequeathed her to me, she was beside herself. She wouldn't look at me, wouldn't sit in my chair, and slammed the door on her way out. I thought I would never see her again.

Volume 19, Number 2: 191–197. March/April 2000.

But she came back and we eventually became friends, or at least friendly enough for her to call about once a week with a new symptom that she was confident was the beginning of her final illness: spots in front of her eyes, a feeling that she was about to have a seizure, an episode of faintness on the subway. I would tell her not to worry. She usually didn't believe me, and sometimes I didn't believe myself. She had more than one unnecessary CT scan, I confess. Her t-cells dropped below normal, she went on AZT, and she waited for the end.

One year passed, two years, three. The end came for almost everyone else, but not for Nancy. The other patients were transients in the waiting room; Nancy was permanent, solid as ever, wondering when the other shoe was going to drop.

"Come on, you can tell me, how long? Just give me a hint," she would ask like clockwork once a month in the clinic. She thought I was holding out on her, and so I was. A lot of scholarly estimates of the median survival time for people with HIV infection were flying around in those days. Coincidentally, they were always about the same as the duration of Nancy's infection. So I left it as "I don't know." She still looked skeptical.

It is probably not at all surprising that of all my sick, complicated patients from that time, the one I really came to dread seeing on Wednesday afternoons was Nancy—healthy Nancy with the incessant barrage of questions that couldn't be answered.

The Second Decade

Now, ten years later, caring for people with AIDS in this country has become a lot like taking care of many Nancys. It's not as sad as it used to be, and people aren't as thin as they used to be, but every year brings an even more intense barrage of complicated questions we don't know how to answer.

The first era of AIDS drew to a close in 1996. Before then, while the other clinics down the hall were operating in the twentieth century, we in the ID (infectious disease) clinic (or the special care clinic, the virology clinic, or any of a dozen other euphemisms) were practicing the medicine of a millennium or two ago, right back to the era of Hippocrates. We had little in the way of treatments; we focused instead on diagnosis, prognosis, doing no harm, and plugging leaky dikes as best we could. Our clinics were drenched in classical tragedy, with overtones of *La Bohème* and *Love Story*. Everyone died in the end—except Nancy.

Everything is different now. More than a dozen drugs are on the market that, used in combination, can work miracles in reversing the complications of AIDS. Sometimes the drugs cause such severe side effects that they can't be used, sometimes they don't work, and sometimes they abruptly stop working. But even though the drugs are far from perfect, AIDS death rates continue to fall, and all of the old AIDS-related infections and malignancies we used to see so much of are becoming rare.

Some researchers predict that the current respite will be brief and the bad old days will return. Others think that the change may be permanent. They wonder if strains of virus that have been exposed to the new drugs may be less fit than they used to be and less able to cause disease. Either way, the epidemic is clearly different. Fewer people are dying of HIV infection, so more people are living with it. Clinics are getting crowded with patients who track their blood tests with the focus and ferocity of hard-core gamblers at the track.

Two of my patients are salesmen—one sells golf clothing at an elegant department store in midtown Manhattan; the other sells T-shirts, stuffed yellow ducks, and a little Xanax (a prescription tranquilizer that is very popular on the streets) out of a shopping bag on the Upper West Side. Both have been taking HIV medication since the early 1990s, adding new drugs one by one as the Food and Drug Administration (FDA) releases them. Now their viruses have been exposed to most of the medications we have and may be resistant to all of them. Both take time from work for their clinic appointments, look at their blood-test results, grimace, and head back to their customers. For three years their blood tests have predicted that they will be getting sick soon. But blood tests may not tell the whole story any more. So far, they both feel fine.

You never know how a person will choose to spend a shore leave of unclear duration. Some patients read nothing but the glossy magazines and drug company–sponsored newsletters now targeted at people with HIV infection and spend their days traveling from one support group to another. Others are going off disability, back to school, or back to work. A few are happily heading back to shooting up and heavy-duty partying. Every last one of them looks me straight in the eye and says all the right things about safer sex, but I've diagnosed two cases of gonorrhea and a case of syphilis in the past four months—a sign that some have thrown all caution to the winds.

Doctors and patients alike, we are all waiting to see what happens next.

Drugs, Striped Fingernails, and Hope

In early 1996 I met a twenty-four-year-old man just released from prison. He looked all too familiar—fragile and feverish, with a big liver, low blood counts, and the peculiar, wide-eyed stare that generally turns into AIDS dementia. This was Mario, a very nice kid with late-stage AIDS. I thought he had a lot of problems. As far as he was concerned, he had only two: He wet his bed occasionally, and his fingernails were turning dark.

I started Mario on a combination of antibiotics, and his swollen liver began to shrink. A neurologist prescribed something to relax his spastic legs, and his walking became a little easier. The social worker got him into a nice nursing home near the hospital.

Then it was time to address his AIDS medications. Permanent dark stripes on the fingernails are a well-known side effect of one of the drugs he was carrying around in his knapsack. It turned out that in an effort to get rid of the stripes, he had quietly stopped taking all of the drugs months before.

I gave him a combination of different drugs to try, and his next clinic visit was like the moment in the movies when the black and white turn to living color and the symphony orchestra begins to play.

Everything was slowly disappearing—the limp, the big belly, the little skinny arms and legs, the incontinence, and even the flaky skin in the middle of his forehead. He gained fifty pounds. He moved out of the nursing home to live with a roommate, then moved again into his own apartment. He decided that it was time to get a job. His discolored fingernails grew out.

In the middle of last year, his blood tests began to deteriorate again. The only combination of drugs left to give him had to include the fingernail-striper. For a few months he stalled. Finally he forced himself to make the switch—and he hasn't looked back since.

Mario finished his job training and his parole. He took a job as a supervisor in the same AIDS day-treatment program where he was once a client. Now he's a stressed-out member of middle management, a harried young executive with striped fingernails. He has his first checkbook and his first furniture. He is speaking to his parents again. He says he may dye his hair red (his mother is against it). His blood count and his liver tests are normal.

Every month Mario comes to see me, leans back in my office chair, and sighs. "Working with the public is so hard," he says. "Especially when they're sick."

Last month he suddenly took off his Walkman headphones—a sign that something serious was on his mind. "I wanted to ask you . . . Do you think I'm ever going to get really, really sick? I mean, am I ever actually going to get AIDS?" There was dead silence as I considered and rejected each of a dozen answers. All I could come up with was, "I sure hope not."

Reality Unacknowledged

I've known Pete for longer than Mario—almost five years now. Until the police cracked down on the vagrants in the Port Authority bus station in New York City, he spent most of his time there, socializing somewhere in the basement. He is more or less illiterate, a little retarded, and a little paranoid, but still extremely charming. He calls me "sweetheart," "darling," or "Mrs. Zuger."

"Sweetheart," he said the day we met, "I really believe that I do not have this virus. I really, really believe that when they had me tested they made a mistake."

I retested him and showed him the results, but since he doesn't read well, seeing something in black and white lacks its usual clout.

"Sweetheart, I really believe, I really, really believe that I am not going to get sick from this virus."

His blood tests showed otherwise. He began to lose weight and feel sick. In the summer of 1996 a committee met to get him started on the new AIDS drugs. We had the health educator, two social workers, two nurses, Pete, me, and the pillbox that beeps at medicine time. The most difficult part of the whole project was getting him to stay home from the Port Authority long enough to let the FedEx man with the drugstore package in the door.

After that it went like clockwork. On a protease inhibitor and a couple of other drugs, his blood counts soared. He said he felt good. Then he began to feel a little too good.

"Darling, I have something I have to tell you. I do not, I do not like being reminded every day about this virus. I really believe that when they did the test, they made a mistake. I would like to talk to the doctor that did the test."

After six months he stopped taking his pills, and no committee has ever been able to put him back together again. I've sent him home a dozen times with new pills; I've called his long-suffering sister, his social worker, a health educator, a psychologist, a psychiatrist, visiting nurses, home health aides. Nothing has worked.

"Sweetheart," he says, "I have to ask you this very serious: Can you make me a tape recording of you, Mrs. Zuger, saying that I have to take these pills, because I will tell you the truth, when I get home I will really believe that when they did the test they made a mistake."

Now he's crashing in slow motion. A few months ago he came in with a fever, a cough, and pneumonia on his chest x-ray. I put him in the hospital where a team of young optimists treated him for everything except the most common AIDS-associated pneumonia, PCP. I realized midway through the second of two frustrating discussions with their leader that PCP is becoming so rare that none of them had ever seen a case before. After the first week Pete decided, not unreasonably, that they were killing him in the hospital, and he eloped for home. His sister dragged him to another hospital where he finally got treated for PCP. He got better.

He came back to the clinic a few months ago very thin and quiet, almost transparent in the waiting room crowd. It used to be that there were only a few solid ones out there, like Nancy, in a sea of ghosts. Now we have one or two ghosts in a sea of regular types. The ghosts are almost invisible, a few bad vibes amid all the good ones, easy to overlook.

Pete accepted some prescriptions, but he missed his next appointment. I called him.

"I threw them all out," he said, "because I really believe, I really, really believe that these were the pills that made me so sick that I had to go into your hospital where they tried to kill me. Now I am doing fine."

I keep meaning to call him again but keep forgetting. Once you get used to a new era, it's hard to go back.

Nancy Today

Nancy spans the old era and the new. She lives down South now but still likes to check in. Her t-cell count is still a little low, although it hasn't changed all that much since 1990. Her feet have started to hurt from one of her medications, and she tells me she thinks she has "lipodystrophy," a disfiguring repositioning of body fat that affects some people with HIV after many years on medications. In the snapshots she sends she does look a little "off," with a new double chin, heavy shoulders, and tiny little toothpick legs.

Otherwise, though, she is healthy. Her son towers over her in the pictures—he used to be a cute little boy who loved to see her get her blood drawn and is now a huge, unrecognizable, unsmiling guy with a mustache, who is about to graduate from high school.

At one time all Nancy wanted was to live long enough to watch him graduate. Then she decided that she might just like to graduate herself. Now she takes college courses, cleans houses for a living, and has been talking about going to nursing school. She used to wonder if she would survive the training. Now she just wonders if she can afford it.

Nancy hates to talk about her illness, which she still thinks of as a terrible stigma. She put off telling her son for a long time. Her big news when she called last week was that years after deciding she wanted to tell her favorite housecleaning client about her HIV, she finally worked up the courage to do it.

"It couldn't have gone better," she said, flying. "The lady was really great." I figured something truly inspirational had occurred.

And it did, although not exactly what one might expect. The client—a retired nurse—managed to come up with what may be the single best way to summarize HIV these days, a phrase that perhaps should replace that tired red ribbon as our mantra for this strange second decade of AIDS:

"Oh," she replied. "OK. See you next week."

∼ The Yellow Baby

A young, uninsured patient falls through the cracks of our medical system.

FITZHUGH MULLAN

When Tim Greene arrived at the clinic, he knew something was wrong because a police cruiser and a rescue squad ambulance were parked askew in front. He loped past apprehensive faces in the waiting room and pushed through the knot of paramedics and office staff

Volume 22, Number 6: 234–238. November/December 2003. This narrative is a short story and its characters are fictional.

at the treatment room door. Inside he found two of his fellow physicians, several nurses, and a paramedic huddled over a small, inert, and very yellow infant. An IV dripped, and multiple electrical leads connected the baby's tiny frame to a monitor. The mood in the room was tense.

Dr. Moreno, gloved and sweating, looked up from the ventilator balloon she pumped rhythmically. "Basically D.O.A.," she said to Greene. "Damn it, we've done everything like clockwork. Everything. But we can't get a pulse back. Look." She pointed to a monitor in the corner of the room showing a series of flat lines. "He's your patient."

The words exploded in him. His patient. *His* patient? This small, yellow, moribund creature was his patient. "Who is he? What happened?"

Setting the balloon down, Moreno looked at her team. "It's been forty-five minutes. We can stop now. Sorry." She leaned against the wall and looked at Greene. "I don't know the whole story, Tim. The baby is two weeks old. Apparently you saw him for a checkup a few days ago. The mother brought him in this morning, jaundiced, bundled, not breathing, a threadbare pulse that disappeared. We never got it back. That's all I know. Babies shouldn't die. Not like this." The nurses turned off the monitor and began removing the electrical leads. *Your patient* is all that Greene could hear. "Is there a chart? When did I see him? Did I know he was sick?"

"Here's what we have." Moreno handed Greene a slim medical file. Baby Cruz, later named José, had been born at the local public hospital fifteen days earlier weighing a respectable eight pounds six ounces and went home two days later with his mother. His hospital stay had been routine, although the discharge note recorded "minimal jaundice" and a minor blood-group incompatibility between mother and child. The record indicated that follow-up care would be at the Valley Health Center. José Cruz's mother had dutifully brought the baby to the clinic for a checkup at ten days of age, and Greene had seen them. Greene remembered José now, a cute, active infant, whose skin was tinged with yellow—a mild jaundice.

Greene also remembered Mrs. Cruz's story, one much like many of the clinic's patients. She had come north to the United States in search of work and without papers. She had no health insurance, no money, and, "illegal" as she was, no Medicaid. The local hospital delivered her with neither enthusiasm nor questions and sent her and her baby to the Valley Health Center, whose mission was caring for the poor and uninsured. Greene, Moreno, and their colleagues treated hundreds of patients like the Cruzes and were well equipped to deal with the basic medical needs of their families—well-child care, respiratory infections, gastroenteritis, diabetes, hypertension, and the like. But things became more complicated when a patient needed something that the health center couldn't provide on site, such as consultations, medications, hospitalizations, and lab tests.

It was a lab test that José Cruz needed at his visit with Greene five days earlier. The blood incompatibility between mother and child was the likely cause of the jaundice. Greene's conclusion at that visit, recorded in the chart and in his memory, was that the baby looked fine but that the jaundice needed to be tracked. Even though Mrs. Cruz didn't qualify for Medicaid, José, an American citizen, did. But making this theory a reality required Mrs. Cruz to present herself at the proper government office with José's birth certificate and evidence of her meager income. It would also take time and patience. Greene did not have time. He filled out the requisition for the lab test, a bilirubin level, as well as a form that would authorize the lab to charge the health center the $75 for the test.

Later that day the lab called Greene to inform him that the bilirubin was 10.5, an elevated level consistent with the baby's hue but not dangerous. Greene reached Mrs. Cruz by phone, explained the test results, and gave her an appointment for José in one week. He told her, however, that if the baby became more jaundiced or showed any signs of decreased feeding or activity, she should bring him back at once. He had not heard from Mrs. Cruz since that phone conversation.

There was pandemonium in the waiting room. Dr. Moreno had informed Mrs. Cruz of the baby's death. She was sobbing in a corner, comforted by several distraught women. The paramedics were packing their gear, and a dozen other patients besieged the receptionist, wanting to know what was happening and when they would be able to see a doctor. Greene needed to talk to Mrs. Cruz for her sake and his. He entered the waiting room with warring emotions raging through him. José was his patient. Greene had only seen him once, but José's little life had been in his hands. "How could this have happened?" he demanded of himself. "How could I have let him die?" Greene watched Mrs. Cruz, disheveled, tear-streaked, empty-handed. "She was the mother," he reminded himself. "She was his source of life, his protector . . . his mother. How could *she* have let him die?"

Mrs. Cruz sat coddled between two large women, crying hard. "I am sorry for what happened," Greene said in fluent Spanish. "I am so sorry." He squatted in front of her and put his hand on her arm. She continued to cry. "They did everything they could for José. Everything medically possible." She said nothing. She continued to weep silently, looking first at Greene and then beyond him. "What happened?" he asked, the inquisitive and the accusative rising together within him. "How did he get so sick?" She shook her head, sobbed, and said nothing. "Why didn't you bring him back to see me?" Greene waited another minute feeling very uncomfortable. He stood. "Mrs. Cruz, I am so very sorry."

Greene had no idea how to deal with the death of the baby. The police came and interviewed everyone, investing the sad scene with a criminal tinge. The baby's body was shipped off to the medical examiner for autopsy, and the health center staff tried to piece together what had happened. Greene himself felt mostly guilt: Why hadn't he ordered a repeat bilirubin or seen the baby back sooner or been sufficiently vigilant to foresee trouble? But his guilt was tempered by an occasional burst of anger: How could she let the baby die? The autopsy report was nonspecific, concluding that the baby's death was caused by heart failure associated with congestion of the lungs. It noted that jaundice was present. The police were satisfied that foul play was not involved and closed the case quickly. The health center staff concluded that their emergency drill had functioned well.

A week after José's death, Greene called Mrs. Cruz and asked if he could see her. She agreed, and that afternoon he climbed down a crumbling, graffiti-ridden stairwell to the basement apartment she shared with relatives. Mrs. Cruz was a small, sturdy woman in her mid-thirties with straight black hair and Mayan features. She wore black and seemed sad but resolute. "Thank you for coming, Doctor."

Greene wanted to know exactly what had happened to the baby but felt intrusive asking directly, so he queried her about herself. "My husband died. We had no work. I left my two older children with my mother and came here to America. I am making money to support them and, maybe, to bring them here with me. I did not mean to start another family, but when I became pregnant I was happy to think that I would have an American family." She talked easily and did not seem angry with Greene. She explained that she had two jobs, one cleaning an office building weeknights from four to midnight. On weekends she spent twelve-hour shifts washing dishes in a Chinese restaurant. She described her work with neither pride nor complaint. Greene asked about her trip north. "Three years ago I left my children. That was hard, but I know they are well cared for." She borrowed all the money she could and started by bus across several borders and through Mexico. She was often molested by men along the way. At the U.S. border she paid a "coyote" three thousand dollars to smuggle her into the country in the back of a garment truck, huddled with five others, surrounded by racks of ball gowns. She used her last money to take a bus north to join her cousin, who found her immediate work. "The work is difficult. I do not speak English and there is no time to learn. But I can make money to send home for the children and save a little to bring them north. It is not a happy life, but I am happy for the future."

Mrs. Cruz knew little about medical care. She had borne her previous two babies at home and had never been to a hospital. When she became pregnant with José, she waited until she was ready to deliver, fearing deportation. "I was surprised," she reported. "Many people in the hospital were nice to me. Some even spoke Spanish. When I went home they told me to go to your clinic with José to get an appointment for his care."

"That's when you came to see me?" asked Greene. She nodded. "Forgive me for raising a difficult topic, but could we talk about José?" Greene paused. "I'd like to know how he got so sick. Could you tell me about it?"

The face of this plain-spoken woman from the Central American countryside darkened a little. "Doctor, José was never a strong baby. Yes, he took the breast and gained some weight, but he was always yellow and weak. After visiting you, I kept feeding him, but soon he began to suck less. I could tell because my breasts were still full when he was done sucking. And he was more yellow." With more of an edge than he intended, Greene asked, "Why didn't you come and see me? Why didn't you bring José in?"

"I did," she replied. "I brought José back as you told me to do. It was in the morning. The clinic was very busy. There wasn't even a place to sit in the waiting room. When I got to the lady at the desk, she didn't speak any Spanish. Another mother translated for me. I told her the baby was sick and needed to see you. The lady said you were too busy and I already had an appointment scheduled with you. I should keep that appointment and if there were problems before that, I should go to the emergency room."

"She said that?" Greene groaned. "She really said that?" Mrs. Cruz nodded. He envisioned the chaotic waiting room on a busy morning and the uncomprehending negligence of the frazzled receptionist. "What did you do?"

"Since I had no money to pay, I waited to go to the emergency room until the next day. The baby was eating very little and the yellow was worse. Then I went. I never saw anybody there but the billing woman, who told me that since I didn't have Medicaid, I needed to go to the Valley Health Center. When I told her that they were too busy to see me, she said that was not her problem. The health center was for patients like me who had no insurance. What she said was wrong, but what could I do? I took José home and gave him the breast, but he hardly sucked. He cried less and was very weak. I tried to give him rice water and put a [good-luck] bandage we call a *fajero* on his stomach. That night his cry was quiet. I knew he was very sick. I knew you had to see him, so in the morning I took him to your clinic the first thing and told the woman I thought he was dying. She took me right in that time."

Greene looked down at the worn, dirty linoleum that covered the floor of Mrs. Cruz's basement. He felt terrible remorse. He had not been vigilant. José had died without his care. What had he been thinking? Had not all his training as a physician taught him that the first weeks of life were the most vulnerable? He should have scheduled José sooner. He should have repeated the bilirubin. He should have figured out that José was sick—blood problems, infection, dehydration, liver disease, meningitis, whatever. Mrs. Cruz watched Greene study the floor. She was sad for José, but she also felt a sadness for this doctor who seemed so upset.

Even as he fretted about his role, he cast about for other explanations for the death—and they were not hard to find. I can't be responsible for everything that goes on, he thought. Where was Medicaid when José needed it? She ought to sue the hospital. They turned her away without so much as an exam. But the ER was not any worse than Greene's own front office, he had to admit. Busy, yes, but murderers? Who was on the desk who knew so little as to turn away a twelve-day-old whom the mother said was sick? Surely the front desk was to blame, or the hospital, or the Medicaid system, or the people in the state capital or Washington, or somewhere. I'm a doctor, Greene thought. I'm not a social worker or a politician. He looked up and saw Mrs. Cruz watching him with resignation. And yes, Mrs. Cruz, he found himself thinking, you're to blame in this. Why were you so polite? Why did you go home when the bureaucrats told you to? You were giving the baby rice water when you should have been banging on the clinic door.

Reflecting on the sturdy, benevolent face of Mrs. Cruz, he recoiled from the meanness of his own thoughts. This woman had traveled thousands of miles to clean floors and wash dishes in a city where Greene lived. She brought her quiet rural customs and personality with her and took her chances with the U.S. medical system. Finally, Greene said, "I don't know exactly why José died, Mrs. Cruz. It could have been a number of things. The autopsy didn't give us the answer. Whatever it was, a lot of people let it happen. José was born in America, and we didn't pay enough attention to him to keep him alive. I am sorry. All I can do is apologize to you—for me and for the others."

She ran her hands over the folds in her long skirt. "Dr. Greene, I know that you tried and that you did not want José to die." A ray of sun shown through the small basement window above her head. "I am a woman, Doctor, and there will be more Josés. Perhaps you will take care of them." Greene felt tired as he climbed the stairs and walked back out into the afternoon light.

⌇ *Blind Faith and Choice*

A blind British health economist and her guide dog meet the realities of choice in the United States.

RHIANNON TUDOR EDWARDS

It was quite a military exercise to get us all—me, my husband, two children (aged nine and five), and my guide dog, Vikki—from Wales to Seattle, Washington, in the fall of 2004. I have retinitis pigmentosa, have been visually impaired since birth, and have been legally blind for the past ten years. Vikki, a black labrador retriever, is my first and only guide dog. I've learned a lot—sometimes inadvertently and often unexpectedly—from her, even about U.S. health care. As I sit and reflect on our time in the U.S., she snores gently at my feet.

As background, I am a health economist from the United Kingdom who spent a year in the U.S. studying U.S. health care thanks to a New York–based foundation that provides fellowships to mid-career scholars from

Volume 24, Number 6: 1624–1628. November/December 2005.

British Commonwealth countries. With its assistance, I spent a year in Seattle at a health studies center. My overwhelming sensation from living in the U.S. is one of bewildering choice. The right to choose and the act of choosing are a national obsession. I was overwhelmed by the heart-stopping, paralyzing choice of coffees (particularly in Seattle, the home of Starbucks), TV channels, and salad dressings—and, of course, the role of choice in U.S. health care.

Traveling with Vikki, my family and I were bemused, amused, and occasionally baffled by such a truly American phenomenon as doggie day care, where you can maintain contact with your pet over the Internet throughout the day. There are hotels that not only tolerate visitors with canine pets but actually supply a range of designer dog biscuits for your four-legged friends and provide dogs to dogless guests craving canine company. Amongst its wide range of restaurants, Seattle is home to the Three Dog Bakery, where owners can take their dogs for brunch.

A Tale of Two Medical Visits

During our time in Seattle Vikki developed a large lump on her side, and we decided to take her to a vet. As we walked into the veterinary office, we were greeted warmly and offered a choice of three vets. On what basis was I supposed to choose amongst these vets, never having met them and not knowing what was wrong with my dog? All I wanted was someone who would look at Vikki, provide any necessary treatment, and reassure me. Then I would be on my way. The lump turned out to be a simple benign tumor that probably resulted from a bite received during a rough-and-tumble play session at an off-leash dog park. Ten minutes and $120 later, the tumor had been drained, and we left reassured. The vet explained that we might have to have it drained again. Because we were on a pretty tight budget, the additional cost of a possible second draining was a real factor in deciding how to manage Vikki's care.

In the U.K. all veterinary costs for guide dogs are covered by the Guide Dogs for the Blind Association. This charitable organization is the single provider of guide dogs for blind people in the U.K. It covers all of the costs associated with guide dog ownership throughout the life of the dog. There is no choice of guide dog providers, but there is universal coverage of the costs associated with owning a dog, which removes any financial barrier to ownership. This is essential, given that 70 percent of blind and visually impaired people of working age in the U.K. are unemployed. That figure is much the same in the U.S. It takes about the same amount of time (six to twelve months) in both countries for a suitable dog to be matched to a blind person. In the U.S., people can choose from a range of guide dog providers all over the country, such as Pilot Dogs, Guiding Eyes for the Blind, Inc., and Guide Dogs of America. However, owners must cover veterinary and other costs of owning a guide dog themselves, either through insurance or out of pocket.

As if in sympathy to Vikki's plight, I developed what can only be described as roaring sinusitis. This is the kind of sinus pain that makes your face ache right down into your teeth. I put up with it for two weeks, consuming copious amounts of over-the-counter decongestants and breathing in steam inhalations. Eventually I decided it was time to consult a doctor. My sponsor offered a pretty comprehensive health insurance package through Blue Cross and Blue Shield. At a time when I wanted nothing more than to curl up in bed, I had to go online to make my way through a bewildering array of acronyms—HMO, PPO, and so on—to find providers covered under our insurance. Once I had chosen one of these providers, I had to select from a range of specialist physicians and specify a geographical location. All this choice at a time when I felt rotten. Once I had located a number of family doctors, I found that none of them could see me for between twenty-four and seventy-two hours, and, worryingly, none would guarantee that they would accept my insurance—despite the fact that I'd located each physician through my health insurer's Web site. The irony was that in the U.S. there was more choice of providers unable to offer me an immediate appointment. In the U.K. it is routine to wait a day or two for a primary care appointment at your nearest general practitioner (GP) clinic. It is possible to choose with which clinic to register; however, in practice, we simply registered with our nearest provider.

Eventually, my husband, Paul, and I elected to go to a family health clinic in Seattle that took walk-in patients. The waiting room was extremely basic, and the bedside manner with which we were greeted was far less friendly than at the vet's office where Vikki was treated. It went through my mind that this visit was not the outcome of an informed choice. The first question put to me was whether I would be billing an insurance company for the appointment. I then had to surrender my insurance card and wait whilst it was checked. The primary concern of the clinic was not "What is the problem?" or "Have you been here before?"—just "How will you be paying?" After handing over my Blue Cross insurance card, I was presented with five pages of forms to complete. The forms asked for background information, Social Security number, insurance details (again), and then there was a health questionnaire. Of course, for a blind or visually impaired person, forms are difficult or impossible, so this became a job for Paul.

After waiting about half an hour, I was asked for my $5 copay. Another half-hour later, I was shown into a small examining room. Fifteen minutes after that, a nurse practitioner came in, confirmed that I had a sinus infection, and wrote a prescription for Augmentin. On the way out, the receptionist—who wanted to photocopy the prescription I had been given—chased us across the road. All of the records, I learned, were paper and kept for only one year. At the Safeway pharmacy I was asked for more insurance details and proof of identity. The pharmacist wanted to see my driver's license, which, as a blind person, I was not able to produce. By now I was feeling really rough. Two signatures and a further $5 copay later, I had the antibiotics in my sweaty little hand and retreated to bed.

In the following week, concerned American friends asked, without exception, what brand of antibiotic I had been prescribed. This just would not happen in the U.K. Perhaps we have a naïve acceptance that antibiotics are antibiotics and that the doctor would have prescribed whatever was appropriate. What is more, we probably don't even consider that we might have had a choice in the matter.

Ice Cream, Health Care, and Choice

The following weekend, on a recuperative visit to Baskin-Robbins, it struck me that although thirty-one flavors of ice cream—a different flavor for each day of the month—are rather overwhelming, I was able to make an informed choice. Of course, since I'm blind, this involved Paul reading aloud the list of flavors: "pistachio almond, chocolate chip cookie dough, nutty coconut . . ." He read at least twenty names before he lost patience.

Can we treat health care like ice cream? Does more choice raise collective society benefit or well-being? I guess it all hinges on whether we have the necessary information with which to choose, actually want to choose, and can influence the organization and quality of health care through exercising our choice.

According to economic theory, ice cream is kept at a socially optimum quality, and individual consumer benefit is maximized, by the act of having each of us choose a favorite flavor. Even if we have not sampled "rocky road" or "raspberry royal dream," we can—or most of you can—see it and imagine what it tastes like. Tiny spoons are provided so that we can have a sample. We can weigh the financial sacrifice of paying for the ice cream versus the benefits of its consumption.

Can we as individual patients really do this for health care, too? And do our individual choices about our own health care lead to the kind of overall health care system that many of us would like to see? In economics, the invisible hand of the competitive market is promoted as the most efficient mechanism for balancing supply and demand for goods and services. The invisible hand does, indeed, work very well for currency and for many consumer goods. In a perfectly competitive market there need to be many buyers and sellers who cannot individually influence price. Consumers need to be fully informed and be the best judges of their own well-being. The good or service needs to be homogeneous, meaning the same thing or standard. For example, dollars are dollars in a currency market. There needs to be free entry into and exit out of the market rather than professional control of who can and who cannot supply a good or service to the market. None of these conditions holds in the case of health care. Yet as interest in consumer-focused health care in the U.S. increases, the market is held up as a means to promote that goal of all goals—consumer (in this case, patient) choice.

How valuable is choice in health care? Does it lead to outstanding population health status or equitable access to necessary health care? Apparently not, when the U.S. is compared internationally.

In the end, given all the choice in the world, as patients we depend on an agency relationship where the doctor is the agent acting in our best interest. We depend on our doctor not only to provide what care we need but also to make the decision as to what that care is. A 2002 Harris Interactive telephone survey of 1,013 U.S. adults, which asked whether they had seen or responded to ratings of hospitals or physicians, found that only 1 percent of respondents had made a decision to change health plans, doctors, or hospitals on the basis of performance evidence. It seems that as isolated individual consumers, particularly at the time when we are ill, we cannot influence the organization or quality of health care through the market. The bottom line: Choice leaves us isolated.

Can Less Offer More?

After a stay in the United States I simply do not believe that more choice is better in health care. It certainly is not a rational alternative to universal coverage or even wider basic health care coverage for all. The market mechanism has not led to high-quality health care in the U.S., even for those with health insurance. There are enormous efforts being made to improve the quality of American health care by developing quality indicators. Some of these, such as the Health Plan Employer Data and Information Set (HEDIS) measures, have evolved to help employers choose health plans for their employees. Yet, ironically, given the escalating costs of providing health benefits, this results in employees' being offered a diminishing choice of plans.

Proponents of consumer-focused health care, and in particular health savings accounts, promise that this will restore choice for the consumer. In fact, these things further isolate the patient, making him or her take greater financial responsibility for health care that, in my view, is disguised as the privilege of choice.

On arriving in the U.S., I believed that most Americans wanted universal health care and that it was only a matter of time until political processes led to wider coverage for the forty-five million Americans who are currently uninsured. I was naïve. I truly found it a surprise to read commentaries in U.S. publications disparaging the poor quality and lack of choice that other countries in the Western world allegedly put up with in the name of universal health care. So if individual consumers cannot influence the quality of health care, and if the majority of the population and stakeholders—such as insurers and providers—do not want a greater role for government in organizing and financing health care, how can the quality of U.S. health care be improved?

The current wisdom appears to be that the key to quality improvement will be through pay-for-performance. This is not a new panacea. All forms of provider reimbursement (fee-for-service, per capita payment, and salary) are in some way paying for performance. What is certain is that however future pay-for-performance schemes are designed, providers will respond and deliver whatever is being paid for, whether or not this leads to better health status or more equitable access to necessary care in the U.S.

Ultimately, choice comes at a price. As consumers, we are expected to pay for the privilege of choice, and if we cannot pay, we do not *get* to choose and, more than likely, do not *get* at all. In the ice cream market, if we can't all afford ice cream every day, it's not a life-or-death situation. With health care, it's very different.

After my year in the U.S. came to an end, my family, Vikki, and I returned to the U.K. having made many American friends and in awe of the natural beauty of the Pacific Northwest. With respect to ice cream and health care, Vikki and I both chose the "rocky road" route. I left the U.S. convinced that having less choice in health care is a price well worth paying for universal coverage.

CHAPTER 4

THE MADDENING SYSTEM

FRUSTRATIONS AND SOLUTIONS

Of Wheelchairs and Managed Care ANDREW I. BATAVIA

Getting the Elderly Their Due DAVID CARLINER

My Mother and the Medical Care Ad-hoc-racy
DAVID M. LAWRENCE

Tin-Cup Medicine FITZHUGH MULLAN

Acquainted with the Night PAUL RAEBURN

Learning Genetics SHARON F. TERRY

∼ Of Wheelchairs and Managed Care

Fighting a system that is loath to finance nonbasic wheelchairs is tough, even for a savvy, Harvard-trained lawyer.

ANDREW I. BATAVIA

After twenty-five years of living with high-level quadriplegia, I was familiar with the routine. Every five or six years my wheelchair-repair person would tell me that my chin-controlled motorized wheelchair (equipped with a recliner system designed to reduce my risk of developing decubitus ulcers) was getting old and could be expected to break down with increasing frequency in the coming year. I would then ask my primary care physician to write a prescription for a new motorized wheelchair using the precise specifications I provided, send the prescription to my insurance company, and prepare for battle. I never looked forward to the kabuki dance that would follow, but I was able to endure it, content in the knowledge that I would ultimately prevail and obtain the wheelchair I needed to maintain my independence and employment.

However, last year the routine changed. I had the same conversation with my wheelchair-repair person. I presented the same list of specifications to my primary care physician, and I was prepared to take my combat position in the epic confrontation with my preferred provider organization (PPO), Blue Cross and Blue Shield (BCBS) of Florida. However, this time I found that the battle lines and alliances had changed. For the first time in my life as a person with a disability, my primary care physician refused to write the prescription. For the first time I was not certain whether I would be able to obtain the wheelchair I needed. More fundamentally, for the first time I asked myself: Is my primary care physician on my side or that of the managed care plan?

Volume 18, Number 6: 177–182. November/December 1999.

My Physician's Position

Before shouting "treason," I decided that rationally I should attempt to learn why my doctor refused to write the prescription or, as I perceived it, refused to open the gate between me and my new wheelchair. I was hoping for a simple, innocuous explanation. For instance, he had already written too many prescriptions that day and was experiencing "prescription burnout" (a new psychiatric diagnosis under the *Diagnostic and Statistical Manual of Mental Disorders*). And if I just came back the following day he would write it. Unfortunately, the situation proved to be far more complicated than that.

When I confronted my physician directly with this issue, he responded that he did not know anything about motorized wheelchairs and that I should talk to his office manager, who had spoken to a BCBS representative. My conversation with the office manager from which I still have not fully recovered, went something like this:

ME: I am very disturbed that Dr. Harris will not write a prescription for my new chair, Ms. Johnson. My current chair is falling apart.

MS. JOHNSON: I spoke with a representative from your PPO, who informed me that they are willing to pay for the repair of your chair but not for a new one.

ME: But each time it needs to be repaired I won't have the use of it. My wheelchair-repair person has informed me that my current chair is at the end of its useful life and breakdowns are likely to become more and more frequent. Every time it breaks down, the effect on me is similar to as if your legs just stopped working. I can't work, I can't pick up my kids from school, and it could be hazardous if the chair breaks down in the middle of a street.

MS. JOHNSON: I am just telling you what your company told me.

ME: Okay, if that's the case, why don't you just give me the prescription and I'll fight it out with the PPO.

MS. JOHNSON: The doctor won't write the prescription for you.

ME: Why not?

MS. JOHNSON: How are we to know if you really need a new chair or if the current chair can still be fixed? If we were to write the prescription and you do not really need a new chair, we could be subject to claims of health care fraud.

ME: I teach health care law. It's extremely unlikely that you would be subject to such claims if you indicate in good faith that I am a quadriplegic with a wheelchair that is more than five years old and in growing disrepair.

MS. JOHNSON: We do not know if the chair can still be fixed.

ME: Any piece of equipment can still be fixed. The question is whether it's worthwhile doing so. Your car could be fixed indefinitely, but you probably wouldn't want to have to rely on it if it were in the repair shop half of the time. How would you get to work? I have the same problem with my wheelchair.

MS. JOHNSON: Do you know how much this new wheelchair will cost? About $24,000. We all end up paying for that. The company has a right to decide whether a new chair is needed or whether the current chair can be repaired.

ME: First, I know how much the chair will cost. It is a highly customized, sophisticated piece of equipment. Do you think I am happy about its price? I'll have to pay about 20 percent of that cost in deductibles and copayments. That's a substantial amount of money out of pocket, and I can assure you that I would not order this chair unless I absolutely needed it. Second, you are right that it is for the company to decide, not you. Now, will you ask Dr. Harris to write the prescription?

MS. JOHNSON: No, I won't. You can have your current chair repaired.

ME: Why do you think you know so much about my chair? How do you know that my chair can still be repaired productively?

MS. JOHNSON: My grandmother is in a similar chair.

ME: Your grandmother must be a high-level quadriplegic. How unusual! There are only a few customized chairs like mine in the country, and she has one of them.

The decibel level of this discourse rose as the discussion grew more and more bizarre. Toward the end it became clear that this doctor's office would not resolve the dilemma.

Why was my primary care physician effectively abandoning me in my effort to get a new wheelchair? Maybe he really believed that writing this prescription without having better knowledge of wheelchairs constituted fraud. More likely, he was afraid to anger the PPO by authorizing an expensive wheelchair that the PPO would have to pay for. Perhaps he was concerned that there would be negative repercussions such as being removed from the provider network, which could affect his livelihood. Whatever the actual reason, I was incredulous that my own primary care physician would not write me a prescription for my wheelchair.

My PPO's Position

My initial theory about why my PPO refused to purchase the new chair related to economics. Although the PPO is willing to pay for repairs, the amount it authorizes for them is quite limited. Moreover, none of the DME (durable medical equipment) preferred providers on its network in my area has the expertise to repair my wheelchair. Therefore, I must pay the difference between the amount charged by my wheelchair-repair person and the amount authorized by the PPO. Because I pay the majority of the repair bill, it is obviously in the interest of the PPO not to pay for a new chair. Its liability for ongoing repairs is relatively small compared with the large cost of a new chair.

On a broader economic issue, many people in the disability community, including me, do not believe that the refusal of health maintenance organizations (HMOs) and other managed care plans to cover the wheelchairs we need is inadvertent. We believe it is part of a strategy to discourage people with disabilities from enrolling in their plans—often referred to as preferred risk selection or skimming. People with disabilities generally have higher-than-average health care costs and are not desirable for an HMO's bottom line. Skimming would be difficult to prove, but it is clear that people with disabilities who require motorized wheelchairs and other disability-oriented services would be foolish to enroll in such plans. Managed care plans surely understand this incentive structure. I had chosen BCBS of Florida as my PPO because it had told me that the company would cover a new wheelchair.

Having analyzed my situation, I then called the BCBS representative to learn the company's position. She indicated that the PPO might be willing to pay for a new wheelchair but that it could not do anything until it received a prescription from my physician. By this time I was beginning to develop conspiracy theories: My physician is unwilling to write a prescription if my PPO is willing to pay to repair the chair, and my PPO is unwilling to pay for a new chair unless my physician is willing to write a prescription for it. A classic Catch-22.

When All Else Fails, Try Another Doc

I was at a temporary impasse. This was not progressing at all according to my plan. I was used to fighting but not to losing. Yet, as an American familiar with the workings of our arcane health care financing system, I had not yet begun to fight. I figured there must be some physician in the network who would be willing to write a prescription for a wheelchair that I obviously needed. This time, I decided not to waste energy with a primary care physician who might repeat the argument that he or she did not know anything about wheelchairs. This time, I sought out a physiatrist—that is, a doctor of physical medicine and rehabilitation.

I duly paid the copayment to speak with a physiatrist in the PPO network. Much to my chagrin, he informed me that he does not have any quadriplegic patients and that those of his patients who use wheelchairs use either manual (nonmotorized) or relatively unsophisticated motorized chairs. Therefore, he did not feel qualified to write the prescription I required. However, after I badgered him persistently (a skill I first developed at Harvard Law School and have since perfected), he eventually agreed to write the prescription.

Which takes longer—ordering a wheelchair or having a baby? After I fought with the PPO for two more months, it finally approved the purchase of the chair. Unfortunately, the PPO approved payment of only $16,000, about two-thirds of the chair's actual cost. No explanation was provided as to how it had reached that figure. I could have contested the allowed amount but by now was tired of this fight and generally satisfied that the PPO had agreed to pay a substantial portion of the chair's price. (This made me better off than other people with significant disabilities who, unlike me, belong to HMOs. I know of no HMOs, with the possible exception of a few social HMOs—which are designed specifically to address the needs of people with disabilities—that would even consider paying for a customized wheelchair such as the one I require. HMOs that cover wheelchairs at all will typically pay for only the most basic chair, which doesn't meet the needs of many disabled people.)

Approval for payment took about nine months from the time of my first inquiry—a gestational period that increased by about four months from the last time I had attempted to purchase a new chair.

The Bigger Picture

My experience suggests that the process for approval of a wheelchair acquisition is at best haphazard and at worst arbitrary. In either case, only the educated, sophisticated consumer is likely to succeed. Others will probably be worn down by the process, and many will simply give up. The cynical among us would argue that this is the purpose of the process.

In developing national and state DME policy, there will be no easy answers. Different individuals have different DME needs and different use patterns. Some will require basic wheelchairs; others, like me, will require customized chairs. Some will need to replace their wheelchairs more often than will others. Some can afford out-of-pocket payments; others cannot. However, the cost of acquiring and maintaining a motorized wheelchair can be extremely burdensome even for someone with a fairly good income. We need to develop a rational process to ensure that all health care payers and managed care plans bear a fair share of the burden in financing wheelchairs and other DME in this country and that they cannot use their coverage and payment policies as a means to discriminate against people with disabilities.

Some analysts might argue that wheelchairs should not even be financed under the health care system, claiming that insurance is intended to protect against risks and that wheelchair costs are certain and predictable. However, wheelchairs have traditionally been financed through health care, and if we are going to change this, we must first develop an alternative source of funding that is reliable and adequate. In the meantime, the current system is inefficient and inequitable from the perspective of both the consumer and the provider. My experience should demonstrate that change is needed.

⁓ Getting the Elderly Their Due

An HMO executive's firsthand view of poor seniors' helplessness in navigating the U.S. health care labyrinth.

DAVID CARLINER

It was a typical call: "Please come over and help me go through my papers." Mrs. Smith complains that she does not understand why she gets so much mail "about the doctors." We promise our members a single place to call for questions, so we respond.

Our Baltimore-based organization, a for-profit Medicare HMO, assists elderly people—overwhelmingly poor and female—in applying for governmental health insurance programs. I accompany a colleague from our sales staff to Mrs. Smith's apartment as part of a program to give senior leaders the chance to witness what other team members do and to see firsthand the impact of our work on an individual level. On a more typical day I sit at my desk, far from the reality of our members' lives, engaged in policy and administrative tasks such as working with the federal and state governments to provide comprehensive services for HMO members.

Overwhelmed and Uninformed

Our visit to Mrs. Smith (not her real name) occurs on a brisk winter day just before spring. Optimism is in the air in most parts of the city, but not in her neighborhood just blocks from my office, where half of the houses are boarded up. Many of the occupied homes are used as bases from which to sell cocaine. Inside this "war zone" is a subsidized senior high-rise that is operated like a fortress. Only after we are inspected are we allowed to enter this safe zone.

Mrs. Smith meets us at the front door, anxiously awaiting our arrival. After decades of manual labor, she shows significant signs of aging. Her torso

Volume 21, Number 6: 198–201. November/December 2002.

is stooped forward, with one hip six inches higher than the other. She looks like a geometric impossibility, like she should not be able to walk. But somehow she does.

We enter her two-room apartment, a combination kitchen/dining room/living room with a separate bedroom and bath. It is quite neat and orderly. We sit at a card table that is covered in papers, grouped and bound by large paper clips and then further aggregated and wrapped in rubber bands. The apparent compulsive organization is a ruse. Medicare Explanation of Benefits forms are mixed in with bills for supplemental policies, housing notices, information from Social Security, from Medicaid—the list goes on. There is no apparent rationale to how the documents are organized; some are current, others decades old.

We begin to sift through them, trying to piece together a story. As we are reading, Mrs. Smith brings over more and more papers. Her filing system is most unusual: Under each cushion on each piece of furniture she stashes additional clipped and banded stacks of papers—thousands of them. How typical is this scene, I wonder? How many other older Americans are bombarded by the unintelligible paperwork that our health care system produces?

We ask a few questions. With each response, we realize that Mrs. Smith does not understand what coverage she has or the programs for which she is eligible but not enrolled in. So we turn to the tangled mess of records to solve the mystery. Like detectives, we look for clues. After considerable study, we have it wrapped.

Mrs. Smith's sole source of income is a monthly Social Security check of $574.27. She has a small bank account with less than $2,000 in it and no other assets to speak of. Somehow for ten years or more she has been paying $150 a month for a Medicare supplemental policy that covers Medicare's deductibles and copayments.

However, she appears to be eligible for the Qualified Medicare Beneficiary (QMB) program—a Medicaid program that pays for Medicare premiums and high copays. Medicare by itself pays for less than 60 percent of total medical costs for a typical beneficiary like Mrs. Smith, making supplemental coverage essential for the poor elderly. QMB, in effect, foots the bill for all of the items covered by her supplemental policy. Like many of her several million peers nationwide, Mrs. Smith is not aware that such a program exists and that it is free. We explain to her that she does not need the Medicare supplemental policy and that she has been wasting $150 a month.

But the story gets worse. Mrs. Smith hasn't been taking her medicines for several months because she needs money for food. Drugs (which Medicare does not cover) also are not covered under her supplemental policy. She could have been using the "wasted" money from that policy for needed medications. Better yet, she is eligible for a state-run drug assistance program that provides prescriptions for a mere $3 copayment (Maryland is one of many states that offer some sort of drug coverage for people like Mrs. Smith). The coverage is free to all who are eligible, but, as for the QMB program, most people don't know they are eligible. Mrs. Smith, like many of our Medicare clients, is dually eligible because her low income qualifies her for Medicaid's QMB program.

People who are dually eligible receive one of the nation's most complete health care benefit packages. Depending on the level of Medicaid assistance for which they are eligible, these persons can have first-dollar coverage for all acute and long-term care services, including access to unlimited drug coverage. Before that can happen, however, the government must find a way to make people like Mrs. Smith aware of their eligibility.

Some 6.7 million Americans are enrolled in both Medicare and some form of Medicaid. But a General Accounting Office report published in April 1999 found that 43 percent of all Medicare beneficiaries who are eligible for Medicare savings programs (what used to be called buy-in programs because the state bought into the program for the beneficiary) are not aware of these programs. A small percentage of these people elect not to obtain Medicaid coverage because of the welfare stigma. However, the vast majority of unenrolled-but-eligible persons simply do not know that the program exists or are intimidated by the application process.

Making a Difference

Action plan for Mrs. Smith: Terminate supplemental coverage immediately. Apply for the QMB and state pharmacy assistance programs. In forty-five minutes we developed a plan to eliminate the $150 a month expense for the supplemental policy and put in motion plans to replace that coverage with free coverage and to get Mrs. Smith coverage for prescription medications.

For the Mrs. Smiths among us, fulfilling an action plan like this one requires great perseverance and know-how. As health care administrators, we understand the system and the various applications that must be completed. But how are lay people—especially the old and infirm—to be expected to navigate the complex, baffling administrative web that we have spun? People have to apply for Medicare and Social Security at local offices of the federally run Social Security Administration (SSA). Two separate applications are required for these programs, and some local SSA offices ask for face-to-face interviews. Medicare beneficiaries have to apply for Medicaid and the various Medicare savings programs at state-operated offices—usually one office will accept applications for both Medicaid and the Medicare savings programs, but not always. Some states require in-person meetings; others allow people to mail in their applications. State application requirements for pharmacy assistance programs run the gamut and often are coordinated by yet another state office. Each of these applications requires extensive documentation that can be extremely difficult for the elderly to produce. Little wonder that so many people are not getting the full advantage of these programs.

Mrs. Smith wept as we left. Although she didn't understand how we were going to do it, she knew that our efforts were going to greatly improve her life.

Another Kind of Reform

The low-income seniors we serve are grateful for everything that we do for them. The social, psychological, medical, and environmental hazards of living a life of poverty take a toll on our clients. They come to us with an average of seven to nine chronic illnesses, which makes caring for them complex.

Mrs. Smith and her peers should know about the programs that augment Medicare, including Medicaid, but they do not. More would if the government were to launch an educational campaign to raise awareness of the interrelationship between Medicare and Medicaid among medical and social service professionals as well as among dually eligible beneficiaries themselves. SSA databases also could facilitate outreach efforts.

States, too, could help more poor elderly persons by streamlining application processes—for instance, by allowing them to apply for federal and state health insurance programs at a single location. The elderly would probably not be as easily scared away if the federal government and states were to develop a shortened, uniform application to assess eligibility for all of these programs. Reforming the application process would go a long way toward ensuring that those in need receive the richest benefits for which they are eligible.

One noteworthy private effort to help seniors understand the public programs for which they are eligible is a Web site created by the National Council on the Aging, www.benefitscheckup.org. Initiatives such as this are a good first step. But Web-based solutions won't reach those who lack computer access, and guidance about eligibility provides only part of the answer for seniors who need help navigating the application process itself.

While our country debates how to modernize Medicare—reforms that will take years—we need to act now to fix the programs that we already have in place. The Mrs. Smiths of America—our mothers, our aunts, our grandmothers—can't do this themselves. They are relying on us.

∽ My Mother and the Medical Care Ad-hoc-racy

The former head of Kaiser Permanente finds that the health care system doesn't work as well as it could, for his mother or anyone else.

David M. Lawrence

It was a phone call children dread. "Mom's fallen," said my sister. "She's in the emergency room at the hospital with a badly broken left leg. Her left shoulder and wrist are broken, too." My mother is an eighty-eight-year-old mentally alert widow who is fiercely independent and lives alone in an eldercare complex. She had tripped and fallen hard while leaving an evening meeting of the Friends of the Columbia River Gorge at a colleague's home in Portland, Oregon. She waited thirty minutes for the ambulance and

Volume 22, Number 2: 238–242. March/April 2003.

several hours in the emergency room before she was admitted for surgical repair of her leg. After a two-hour operation to knit together the three fragments of her femur just below the hip joint, she remained in the hospital three and a half days. She was then transferred to a private skilled nursing facility (SNF) to receive the intensive physical therapy that would enable her to resume her busy life.

A Complex Web of Care

In the first month of her combined hospital and nursing home stay, Mom was cared for by ten physicians: three primary care physicians, an emergency room doctor, two radiologists, an orthopedic surgeon, an anesthesiologist, a geriatrician at the SNF, and a wound care specialist. She was attended by at least fifty different nurses, ten physical and occupational therapists, and a host of nurse aides. Four nurses and two social workers arranged her transfer from the hospital to the SNF; two more arranged her stay in the assisted living section of her eldercare complex. At the SNF the nurse aides who bathed her, helped her with her toilet, and answered her questions were from Ethiopia, Eritrea, El Salvador, Brazil, Cambodia, and Vietnam. Mom had a hard time communicating with this array of nonnative English speakers.

The hospital has a computerized medical records system for inpatient care, but records had to be printed out and hand-carried to the SNF. Because she'd been given blood thinners to prevent clots after surgery, at the SNF Mom bled from an unhealed surgical wound on her right foot each time she tried to do physical therapy. Her dermatologist had removed a cancerous growth at the wound site several months earlier. He was on vacation, though, and his records were inaccessible. Eventually Mom was transported by ambulance across the city to a wound care clinic. The specialist there discovered that the treatment regimen prescribed by her dermatologist was out-of-date and had retarded the healing process. By the time proper treatment began, she'd suffered several months of unnecessary aggravation and lost more than a week of physical therapy at a critical time in her recovery process.

As a result, entirely counter to her usual optimistic nature, she'd also developed frustration and cynicism about the health care system. Mom usually gives the benefit of the doubt to those around her. She was, in fact, happy with her individual providers and felt that, with a few exceptions, her personal needs were well met. What upset her were the mixed signals, the delays, the unexplained changes in treatment plans and prognosis, and the uncertainty about when she could leave the SNF to return to her eldercare facility.

Now, five months after the accident, Mom has moved back to her apartment. She gets around with a walker, does regular physical therapy, but still has the open wound on her foot that requires daily care. Her spirits are good, and she continues to actively participate in the lives of her friends and large family. But the care process was bumpy and poorly organized; the chances for medical error were great; and the costs to our family, Mom's caregivers, and her insurers were far higher than they needed to be.

Too Many Opportunities for Disaster

At times Mom's care seemed like a pick-up soccer game in which the participants were playing together for the first time, didn't know each other's names, and wore earmuffs so they couldn't hear one another. Her care seemed like an "ad-hoc-racy" that involved well-trained and well-intentioned people, state-of-the-art facilities, and remarkable technologies—but was not joined into a coherent whole for the benefit of her or her family. My mother ricocheted from place to place like a pinball. Each contact brought another bill, different advice, and increased risk that something could go wrong. In spite of my experience as the leader of a large integrated health care system, there was little I could do to control what happened to her.

The glitches were many. A part-time physical therapist insisted that Mom could walk on her one-week postsurgical leg, in spite of clear orders to the contrary from the orthopedic surgeon. An occupational therapist told Mom to undo her shoulder and wrist straps in order to "slip into a nice nightgown." Luckily, Mom is mentally alert, irascible, and tough as nails. She quickly sent these caregivers scurrying to check the medical records for proper guidance. Nurses disagreed about how to give her heparin injections and openly criticized one another in Mom's presence. Frequent disagreements among doctors about treatment choices caused her anxiety and confusion. Reflecting on the care process, I would like to offer suggestions for how the system could be improved for everyone, including my mother during her next medical event.

Ways to Do Better

Medicine today, especially emergency, complex, and chronic care, involves large numbers of professionals. Just look at the number of caregivers helping Mom for an acute, though relatively simple, problem! Gone is the day when a single doctor could take care of us. Mom's care would have been quite different had her caregivers acted in well-developed, tightly coordinated teams instead of as an ad hoc collection of individual actors. Instead of multiple opinions about treatment, there would have been one; instead of delays and confusion about changes in treatment, there would have been a clear process for group meetings and decision making. Instead of conflicts among caregivers, there would have been agreement about the role each plays depending on competence, experience, and training. Instead of lost information or miscommunication, there would have been tools for continuous discussion and information sharing. Instead of dropped balls as Mom moved from one care site to the next, there would have been well-designed hand-offs to ensure continuity.

Besides a lack of coordination among providers, I witnessed firsthand a wide variation in individual physician practices. This created confusion for all involved. It also greatly increased the chances that miscommunication and errors would occur, and it raised care costs as well. Expecting caregivers to manage so many different approaches is a recipe for disaster: There's too much to remember and too many differences to accommodate. Each professional caring for Mom had his or her own way of doing things. The dermatologist and the wound care specialist approached the treatment of her foot wound differently. The primary care physician strapped Mom's wrist and shoulder; the orthopedist thought this was overkill. The primary care physician prescribed blood thinners, inhibiting the ability of the physical therapists to provide the therapy Mom required to speed her recovery.

The "gold standard" that obviates these problems is evidence-based care, meaning care that is based on the best medical science now available. The process of deciding what the evidence supports is far from simple; professionals will disagree, the evidence is not always compelling, and judgments must be made to set the acceptable range of choices that the evidence supports. But the rewards of doing so—greater coherence in care and the chance to simplify an overwhelmingly complex process—are worthwhile.

Evidenced-based medicine is the only route to reducing medical errors and providing consistently better, more responsive care.

Some Easily Made Improvements

Sometimes fairly simple changes to the system can be just as important as the more complicated ones. Mom's social and educational supports and her ability to manage her own care have been as critical to her recovery as the medical care she received. Yet the system provided precious little help beyond the medical component of her care. Had her treatment plan included medical, social, and educational interventions and been carefully designed to help her and us manage her care, we would not have been forced to address these needs on our own. Her recovery would have been expedited and her independence bolstered. Understanding Mom's medical treatment and prognosis has been difficult enough. Understanding how to make her apartment safer, manage her reduced independence, and ensure that her ongoing self-care is appropriate has been more challenging still. We've been on our own for the most part, making it up as we go. Here and there people have provided names or contacts. But we've mainly relied on friends, eldercare community contacts, and trial and error. In this, my mother is lucky: Not all patients have the wherewithal, including the family advocates, to do this.

Another comparatively simple, logical improvement to the system that would bring large payoffs would be to automate clinical records. Providers noted critical information about Mom by hand; her paper records were hand-carried by couriers among health care facilities. The large number of caregivers involved in Mom's care, the range of problems faced in returning her to a full life, and the quantity of information to manage in the process underscored for me the limits of traditional information management. The costs and dangers of relying on paper records, informal face-to-face information sharing, phone, and faxes are unacceptably high.

Finally—and maybe this is a harder problem to fix—while careening from caregiver to caregiver and site to site, we felt that no one but us could see the whole process of Mom's problem unfolding. An organization needs to design and manage the care process from start to finish. The individual elements of care that my mother received were generally satisfactory, but the pieces didn't fit together very well. The weak integration across providers and sites produced most of the confusion, delays, dead ends, and higher costs that we experienced. From our perspective, it didn't matter who gave the care or where it was given, so we had difficulty understanding why the left hand didn't know what the right was doing, why information generated in one part of the system wasn't available to another part, and why recommendations differed from stop to stop. The stress generated by this situation was significant for all of us, especially for Mom.

We are grateful for the care Mom received. With the exception of the wound care recommended by her dermatologist, the quality and compassion of her individual caregivers were exemplary. But her care could have been far better for everyone involved. If we could implement some of the changes above, we could accelerate the slow, painful process of transforming a technically sophisticated but poorly organized and wasteful system to one that can bring the remarkable capabilities of modern medicine to patients. If care had been given this way to Mom, she probably would have recovered faster and had more confidence in her caregivers and in her ability to help herself. Her care would have been less expensive for Medicare, her Medigap insurer, and our family. Most important, we all could have focused more on helping Mom return to her active life than on dealing with the problems created by the care system itself.

⌒ *Tin-Cup Medicine*

Resourcefulness, patience, and a willingness to beg are key to practicing medicine on the "safety net."

FITZHUGH MULLAN

Shirley Laotsi is a patient of mine—a big, shy, affable girl who arrived in Washington, D.C., from central Africa two years ago with her refugee parents. Shirley shows no external scars from the long and dangerous journey that took her through several African countries and across the Atlantic. She is in school, has friends, loves television, and is growing

Volume 20, Number 6: 216–221. November/December 2001.

well—too well. Although she has just celebrated her eighth birthday, she shows signs of advancing puberty and has grown quickly to the height and weight of an average twelve-year-old. This pattern of growth is problematic and raises concerns about tumors or endocrine diseases. Even if these possibilities are ruled out, Shirley faces a heightened risk of diabetes and likely social problems. Her rapid growth calls for a series of hormone tests, x-rays, ultrasounds, and a consultation with an endocrine specialist. Lacking work permits, jobs, and medical insurance, the Laotsis have relied on whatever charitable or governmental services are available. They get their medical care at the Upper Cardozo Community Health Center, where I work.

Upper Cardozo is a spacious, unattractive, four-story bunker constructed in the early 1970s when the federal Community Health Center (CHC) program was still building clinical facilities. An African-American neighborhood at that time, the community is now heavily Salvadoran with a mix of other Latino groups, Vietnamese, Africans, and African Americans. Refugees from a variety of nations seek care at our clinic because of its open-door policy and sliding fee scale. The clinic runs special programs for food (WIC), HIV/AIDS, the homeless, and social services. Staff members speak English, Spanish, Vietnamese, Chinese, French, and Amharic. About a third of our patients have Medicaid. The rest, with few exceptions, have subsistence employment at best, no health insurance, and few financial reserves to cover medical costs.

Upper Cardozo is a strand—a thick cord, actually, compared with many of the filaments that make up the amalgam of health care possibilities for the poor and uninsured that we have come to call the "safety net." Upper Cardozo is one of about a thousand community clinics that make ends meet with funds provided annually by the federal CHC program, smaller public and private grants, Medicaid reimbursements, and the tin cup. By the tin cup, I don't mean charity events and fund-raisers (although they have a potential role), but rather, the perpetual, frustrating, quixotic, creative, and demeaning process of begging for services from others for our patients.

We needed the tin cup for Shirley. Upper Cardozo provided her with a pediatrician, some basic blood tests, and the diagnosis of precocious puberty. But then we needed help: special tests and a specialty consultation. A local hospital offers free consultations to a limited number of uninsured patients from health centers such as ours. Our social worker helped the family fill out the many forms required by the hospital; I called the endocrine department myself to make her the appointment. A week later I received a distress call from Shirley's father on a pay phone reporting that the hospital required a down payment of $200 before Shirley could be seen. I then spent twenty minutes talking to voice mail and an occasional person at the hospital clinic, the finance office, and the president's office—which resulted in Shirley's being seen that morning without a deposit. The endocrinologist was good enough to call me with her findings that Shirley's growth was probably a normal variant not caused by a tumor. But the doctor wanted to see her again after more tests, presaging another round of tin-cup challenges.

The Limits of What We Can Do Alone

President Bush has had kind things to say about CHCs, and his 2002 budget proposes increased health center funding. I applaud this initiative, but if he thinks that a few more health centers will fix the safety net, he underestimates the problems. CHCs bring crucial facilities to poor neighborhoods; they bring doctors, nurses, primary care, and urgent care. Since their introduction as part of the War on Poverty thirty-five years ago, they have been central to serving the poor and uninsured. What we do at Upper Cardozo is first rate. We provide basic medical treatments and preventive services and do it in a way that is, for the most part, creative and responsive to the community. In pediatrics we talk the patients' languages. We provide them with immunizations, lead poisoning and anemia screening, two children's books per visit, occasional home visits, and a special clinic for teenagers. Trouble develops, however, as soon as something more is needed—something as simple as a medication or an x-ray. Things quickly get more difficult if we need a specialty consultation, a nonroutine diagnostic procedure, surgery, or hospitalization.

For the minority of our patients who have Medicaid, the problems resolve themselves quickly and usually satisfactorily. Medicaid (even managed Medicaid, which is predominant at Cardozo) covers medications, diagnostic tests, and the costs of specialists and hospitalizations. But for the two-thirds of our patients without Medicaid, the only answer is the tin cup. This means resorting to charity services, give-away programs, personal connections, system loopholes, solicited forbearance, and persuasion.

Getting Vangie Her Due

Vangie Thomas should have had Medicaid but didn't. A sullen, pretty five-year-old, she arrived in the clinic one day with her foster mother and a case of ringworm—a skin infection easily treated with about twenty dollars' worth of medication. Her foster mother, Mrs. McCarthy, an elderly woman with four other foster children, handed me a folder with the official papers accumulated over six months of caring for Vangie. It contained an array of forms, documents, and stubs from several government and intermediary child protective organizations. The central document, as far as I could tell, transferring Vangie to Mrs. McCarthy, was only partially filled out, in longhand, and listed Vangie's names as "Vangie," "Angie," "Thomas," "Promis," and "Thoms." I was satisfied that my little patient's name was, in fact, Vangie Thomas, because the file did contain a photocopy of her Social Security card. What it did not contain was a Medicaid card or any reference to Medicaid.

What kind of system, I asked myself, turned a child over to a foster mother with five versions of her name and no Medicaid card? I began by calling a name and number scribbled on a piece of paper that Mrs. McCarthy told me was her caseworker. Three voice-mail messages and two agencies later, I reached a human being who acknowledged that as a foster care child, Vangie should have Medicaid and agreed to start the process. She assured me that the card would be retroactive. But that would be of no use at the pharmacy that morning. Fortunately, we had a tube of the antifungal medicine Vangie needed and gave it to her. When Vangie returned for a follow-up visit, her infection was improving, and a call to the caseworker produced a Medicaid number—although the worker said she had "no idea" when the actual card might arrive. Happily, the number did work at the local pharmacy for her medication refill, but Vangie would have to be counted as partially insured, a beneficiary of the Medicaid system when and if the multiple agents of child welfare were at their desks and engaged. Banging the tin cup succeeded in getting Vangie tentatively into the system.

An Island of Security

The more severe the problems or the larger the family, the more important Medicaid becomes. At the end of a rainy morning, Mrs. Castro arrived at the clinic with five sets of school immunization forms, one for each of her school-age children. She had four younger ones at home. I knew the Castros well, although I never could keep the children sorted out. They were a blur of illnesses in the clinic, in the hospital, in strollers, on foot, underfoot. We had hospitalized one or another for asthma, diarrhea, and pneumonia. We had treated others in the clinic for rat bite, speech delays, ear infections, anemia, and scores of immunizations.

With the children's charts and the help of a nurse, I filled in the immunization records five times over, the sort of repetitious task that must occupy most of Mrs. Castro's waking hours. At the lunch hour, when we were done, I drove Mrs. Castro home to an apartment that consisted of a corridor that ran the length of the narrow basement of a row house, ending in a kitchen at the back. The apartment walls were bare, the linoleum threadbare, and the cockroaches defiant. School was closed because of a storm warning, and all nine children were milling around, with Mr. Castro as babysitter. When we entered, the younger children ran off with my stethoscope while the older ones showed off gymnastics on the bunk beds. After a brief chat with Mr. Castro, I collected my stethoscope, picked my way through playful children, and retreated to the car.

Life in the Castro family was a sea of chaos in the middle of which was an island of security. Despite poverty and the challenges of a large family, I never needed to use the tin cup for the Castros. The family had health insurance that covered every clinic visit, medication, hospitalization, and consultation. They had Medicaid.

Because of Medicaid, we have the luxury of using the tin cup a bit less in pediatrics than do our colleagues who work with adults. Underfunded as it might be and unpopular as it is in some quarters of the medical profession, Medicaid connects a patient to medications, diagnostic tests, consultants, and hospitals in a way the tin cup never can. The advent of the State Children's Health Insurance Program (SCHIP), in particular, has made Medicaid more available to low-income children. Little by little many more of the kids I see are getting enrolled, although immigrants, refugees, older children, children from disorganized families, and parents still don't get covered. Enrollment can be slow, bureaucratic, and temporary, but Medicaid makes a huge difference in what I can do for children.

Rattling the Tin Cup for the Rest

Without Medicaid, the tin cup comes out as soon as we reach the limits of what we can personally do for the uninsured patient at a health center—the child with a fever and cough who needs a chest x-ray, the diabetic who needs insulin, the teenager with depression who needs Prozac, or the four-year-old with garbled language who needs speech therapy. The telephone figures prominently in tin-cup medicine. I call local agencies to find charitable funds for medications, I call for special openings for speech therapy or mental health exams, I phone specialists or dentists who might see a patient for free. I also write letters: to schools pleading for special education placement, to drug companies begging for medications, or to other physicians asking for opinions. Some days I spend as much time pleading as I do practicing.

Medications are the most predictable and frequent stumbling block in a safety-net practice. Dignity, trust, and momentary circumstance all come into play at the end of an office visit when I ask an uninsured patient if she thinks she can afford the prescription I have just written. I never know exactly what the medication will cost, but I can be sure that it will severely tax a small budget. The clinic purchases and distributes a small supply of basic medications in emergency situations. We also have some samples to distribute, although they rarely meet the need for the precise medication indicated, nor are they available in adequate quantity. Drug company representatives are infrequent visitors to our clinic.

These tin-cup problems are compounded for those who care for adults. Lives can be improved and saved with well-established, relatively inexpensive treatments for chronic, common conditions such as heart disease, thyroid disease, diabetes, and hypertension. The treatments, though, have to be as chronic and persistent as the diseases. Yet since so few adults at Upper Cardozo have any coverage for medications or referrals, the tin cup—with all of its inadequacies—is always in play and rarely sufficient.

Retiring the Outstretched Palm

Medicaid and community health centers are complementary strands of the safety net, running across and reinforcing each other, making the net stronger and more durable. CHCs are extraordinary institutions that provide service to people in need and represent our civility as a society. They put a front line of doctors, nurses, and social workers in communities where they would not otherwise be. But they can't do the job alone. Insurance coverage is a must for a patient to be able to buy his or her way into the rest of the health care system. Medicaid provides that access for health center patients who are fortunate enough to have it. But what about the majority at our clinic, who don't? The tin cup is archaic and inefficient. Expanded coverage for children under SCHIP dramatizes what can be done. Extending coverage to SCHIP parents has been proposed, as have other Medicaid expansions. Lowering the age of Medicare eligibility has been considered in the past as a method of closing the gap for the uninsured, as has a mandate to employers to provide private insurance.

As a tin-cup provider, I salute the president's support for CHCs. But I want to know where he intends to go from here. As he contemplates costly strategies such as doubling the budget of the National Institutes of Health or providing a prescription drug benefit to Medicare recipients, he needs to reflect on fairness in America. If we are serious about putting a floor and not just a net under health care, we will need both more CHCs and expanded insurance coverage to close the health care gap between the poor and the rest of us.

We need to retire the tin cup as soon as possible.

⌒ *Acquainted with the Night*

A father finds sparse institutional support in his quest for appropriate treatment for his mentally ill son.

Paul Raeburn

It's early evening, Tuesday, May 7, 1996, and I am coming home from my job as an editor at *BusinessWeek*. As I enter the house I hear my son, Alex, then eleven years old, screaming at his mother. He is being treated with Ritalin by a psychiatrist who diagnosed him with ADHD (attention deficit/

Volume 23, Number 6: 200–205. November/December 2004.

hyperactivity disorder) after a single fifteen-minute interview. The Ritalin hasn't been working, and the psychiatrist has increased the dose. But Alex isn't reacting well. He's suddenly much, much worse. I try to talk to him, to calm him, but it doesn't work. He only becomes angrier. He says he is going to grab a knife from the kitchen and kill himself. "Where can I hide the kitchen knives?" I think to myself. "What about my shaver? The scissors? The box cutter, paint scrapers, and saws in the basement?" I do the only thing I can think of. I call the psychiatrist back to say we are in trouble. We have an emergency on our hands.

A woman answers. The doctor is not available, she says. You can call back in the morning. "This is an emergency," I say. "My son is threatening to kill himself, and I can't hide all the knives. You've got to tell the psychiatrist what's happening here. We don't know where else to turn." Well, perhaps, she says. "I'll see what I can do."

We wait, watching Alex, the telephone, and the clock. The psychiatrist has given us a sedative for Alex. I grab one of the pills and a glass of water and try to hand them to Alex, explaining that this will make him feel better. He tries to knock the glass out of my hand. Ten minutes pass, or fifteen, or twenty; it feels like hours. The phone rings. It's the psychiatrist. I explain what's happening. "Call the police," he says. "There is nothing I can do for him."

"Can you hear him screaming?" I ask. "The police won't know what to do. You're his doctor. I need help from you." If we call the police, they will take him to the county hospital for mentally ill kids. The hospital has just been the focus of a series of newspaper articles pointing out its lack of supervision and the unusually high rate of suicide among its patients. I'm determined to keep Alex out of that place. But if the psychiatrist won't help, I might not have a choice.

A doctor I've met through a friend has told me that if I want to get the proper help for Alex, I'm going to have to fight for it. This seems like the time to start. "If anything happens to Alex," I tell the psychiatrist, my voice shaking with rage, "I will make it very clear that I talked to you and you refused to help. Alex is out of control. He won't take the medicine you gave us. You've got to do something."

"Let me see," he says. "I'll call you back." An hour later he calls to say that he thinks he can find a hospital bed for Alex in the morning. We will have to get him to take the sedative or watch him all night. There is nothing he can do in the meantime. Alex, who earlier seemed possessed of inexhaustible energy, begins to tire. I try the sedative once more, and he takes it. A few minutes later, he is asleep.

Adding Insult to Injury

When Alex fell ill, I entered part of the national health care system in which nearly everything is broken. For the parents of children with mental illnesses, there is nowhere to turn. They can't find emergency psychiatric care, their insurance companies desert them, they can't find a competent child psychiatrist or can't afford one if they do, and schools deny any responsibility to help. According to the U.S. Surgeon General's 1999 report on mental health, about one in five children and adolescents has a psychiatric illness, and some 5 percent (three to four million) have illnesses so serious that the children suffer "extreme functional impairment." But they are not the only ones who suffer. Millions of parents and brothers and sisters also suffer. Childhood mental illness is an epidemic in this country, one we rarely acknowledge.

The morning after Alex's crisis, the psychiatrist found Alex a bed in a hospital an hour and a half away from our home. The hospital asked for the name of our insurance company so it could arrange to have the admission precertified for coverage. The insurance company said that it could precertify the admission only if the hospital would explain the reason for the hospitalization and why Alex could not be treated as an outpatient. No one at the hospital had even seen Alex or heard his name until that morning, so the hospital could not possibly provide that information. I made repeated calls to arrange for the psychiatrist to provide the information. Even then, the insurance company would not promise to cover the hospital stay until Alex had been admitted and examined at the hospital. We took a chance that we might be responsible for nearly $2,000 a day in charges ourselves if the insurance company refused to pay. All of this was happening less than two weeks after Alex had been discharged from another psychiatric hospital. He had spent a week there, had been examined by a psychiatrist and a neurologist, and had not been given a diagnosis. No one could say what was wrong.

At the new hospital we waited for a tense half-hour before a hospital staff member escorted us to the teenage unit, where Alex would stay until a bed opened up on the children's unit. On the way he became increasingly agitated. "Take me home!" he yelled. Two white-coated aides grabbed him. He told them that his mother and I were making up stories about what he'd done. They half-carried him to the quiet room and locked him inside. I could hear Alex banging against the door and the walls. The hospital staff assured us that they would take over and that Alex would be fine, and they pointed his mother and me toward the door. There was nothing we could do, no reason to stay. Get in the car and go home, they said. As we walked down a long empty corridor, Alex's agonized screams echoed off the walls. I could hear them until we reached the end of the corridor and walked through a large double door. I can hear them still. We finally had taken Alex to a place where he could get care, and their reaction was to lock him up.

When Alex was released, he went back to his elementary school, where the principal, his counselor, and teachers shook their heads. "We've never seen a child like this," they said. "We don't know what to do." Every time Alex was involved in a routine violation of school rules, even if he was late to class, his counselor called home and asked what to do. "Do what you have to," I said. "Just because he's sick doesn't mean the rules don't apply to him. If he deserves detention, give him detention. If he needs a time out in your office, fine." I couldn't be there in the classroom to advise them every minute. While Alex was in school, they would have to exercise their judgment. If he had a serious crisis and appeared to be getting sick, then, of course, they should call me. The truth was that the school wanted to get rid of Alex. Of course they had seen many children before with emotional disorders. With 5 percent of kids suffering from severe mental illness, they had to have seen them. Yet they did nothing to help, except to suggest, from time to time, that Alex might be better off if he were sent away somewhere, to a special school.

Alex saw six psychiatrists over three years before I found one who diagnosed him and treated him correctly. The first one saw him for fifteen minutes and prescribed an antidepressant, which appeared to be responsible for a manic episode Alex suffered a couple of days later, sending him to the hospital. The second one talked to Alex for fifteen minutes, again, and prescribed Ritalin. Another manic episode followed, and another hospitalization. Each time Alex was admitted to the hospital, the insurance company allowed him to stay about six to seven days. Each stay included a weekend, at which time the therapists and psychiatrists were not available for treatment. As a result, during each hospitalization he saw a psychiatrist once or twice, saw a therapist or social worker three or four times, and was started on medication, a different one with each hospitalization. The bill for that meager care? About $10,000 for each week's stay.

Alex was still in crisis, and we were still searching for a diagnosis when, by chance, I discovered that my daughter, Alicia, who was two and a half years younger than Alex, had twice tried to commit suicide, once with a handful of Tylenol tablets and once with Advil. I didn't know it then, but for weeks she had been attacked by the "popular" girls in the sixth grade. They were spreading the story that Alicia had been sexually involved with dozens of boys in their class. It started when Alicia was spotted kissing one of their boyfriends. "Alicia is a slut," they were saying. It's the kind of thing that happens in the sixth grade. The more Alicia protested that she was not a slut, the more the label stuck. Her friends were deserting her. School was becoming unbearable, every day a new trial. The pills were her way out, the only thing she could think of.

Where were her teachers? Didn't anyone see that Alicia was tense in class or unable to do her work? Maybe I expected too much of them. Alicia's suicide attempts did not succeed. Once we knew she was in trouble, we began the years-long process, once again, of finding appropriate diagnosis and treatment. But she might have succeeded in her suicide attempts; many children do. Can we not ask teachers to simply let parents know if they suspect there is a problem?

More Action, Fewer Reports

Since those experiences with Alex and Alicia, I have talked to many other parents in similar circumstances. They want to know where to go for help, how to get their children a proper diagnosis and treatment, and how to coerce stingy insurance companies to pay for it. After eight years of involvement with the medical establishment, the insurance industry, schools, and social service agencies, I'm not sure I've found the answers. I am a writer and a reporter and have spent most of my career covering science and medicine, yet I am struggling. What is the chance that parents without access to the nation's top doctors or who don't know where to go for information will find help? Also, I have the money to pay for care not covered by my insurance company. I've spent tens of thousands of dollars for psychiatric care that wasn't reimbursed. My insurance company has refused to cover the care or would not provide resources of its own.

I have learned a few things from my reporting. As a National Advisory Mental Health Council report concluded in May 2001, "No other illnesses damage so many children so seriously." Many other reports have come to similar conclusions, including that of the New Freedom Commission on Mental Health. It's now gathering dust along with scores of other reports. Next year, or the year after, some well-meaning researchers, parents, community advocates, and psychiatrists will gather to produce another report, and they will conclude the same things.

What can we do to change this? For one thing, parents can speak out. This is not only an epidemic, it's a hidden epidemic. Why? Because we parents are afraid to admit that our children are suffering from mental illnesses. The guilt that parents experience is overwhelming: To the extent that these disorders are genetic, it is our genes that caused them. And to the extent that these disorders are the product of stress at home or at school, we are guilty again—we provided the environment. It's time for us to overcome our reticence, embarrassment, and guilt. As parents, we must speak out, demanding better care for our children. The AIDS activists and breast cancer coalitions offer us a model. They marched in the streets, carried signs, went to Congress, and demanded action. We need to do the same.

We can ask the schools to do more. The American Academy of Pediatrics has called for school-based mental health services. And without putting undue burden on teachers and schools, we can ask that they alert parents when they suspect that a child might be having an emotional problem. Teachers see thousands of children over the course of their careers. With just the least bit of sensitivity, they should often be able to recognize problems before parents do.

We need to provide psychiatric training for pediatricians and family practitioners, who prescribe most of the antidepressant drugs in this country. A single rotation through psychiatry in medical school a decade or two ago is not enough, and some doctors lack even that. These problems are too important to be left in the hands of doctors whose principal source of information may be drug company sales people. We need more child psychiatrists. There are only 7,000 in the country now. Few children with psychiatric disorders will ever see a child psychiatrist. I've asked child psychiatrists why they don't do a better job recruiting; they say they don't know. We also need to improve child psychiatrists' training. There is no excuse for prescribing a potentially dangerous drug on the basis of a short interview, as happened repeatedly with my children. And we need health insurance that provides as much coverage for mental illnesses as it does for any other illness. Congress and the White House have expressed overwhelming support for mental health parity, but congressional leaders do not act on the legislation that would establish it. The reason is that insurance companies and large employers are lobbying ferociously behind the scenes to prevent it.

My kids need help, and so do millions of others. We've had enough reports, enough study, enough examination of the problem. It's time for action.

⌒ *Learning Genetics*

Finding sparse, uncoordinated research on their children's rare disease, a couple starts their own organization to jumpstart hopes for the future.

SHARON F. TERRY

In 1994 we didn't know a gene from a hubcap. We thought we didn't need to know. The brave new world of genetics was vaguely interesting but not part of our world—not until our children were diagnosed with a rare genetic condition and we were thrown headlong into a chasm. The chasm was really a threshold. We crossed it, abandoning our ignorance of medical research and clinical treatments for the other side—a desperate need for those systems to perform exceptionally well. The leap across that threshold took seconds, but learning the realities of these systems was an arduous, eye-opening journey that led us to start a foundation and a new model for accelerating research.

Our children, Elizabeth and Ian, now ages fifteen and thirteen, have pseudoxanthoma elasticum (PXE), a rare genetic condition that causes vision loss, premature wrinkling, and cardiovascular and gastrointestinal dis-

Volume 22, Number 5: 166–171. September/October 2003.

ease. The condition's worst complication is vision loss, devastating people with PXE when they are between thirty and forty.

Two days before Christmas 1994, I brought Elizabeth, then age seven, to a dermatologist. She had small bumps on the sides of her neck that had not disappeared since I had first spotted them a year before. Our pediatrician didn't think they warranted attention and assumed that my worry was spurred by the recent death of my brother from a brain tumor.

The dermatologist knew immediately that these bumps were a sign of PXE. Glancing at Ian, then five, he said, "Ah, he has it too." He asked if he could biopsy Elizabeth's neck and examine her eyes. Confused and terrified, I consented. Why would a dermatologist examine eyes for a skin condition? I learned all too quickly that many skin problems are part of larger, systemic conditions. I also learned that we were fortunate that the dermatologist we chose, who happened to be a neighbor, also happened to be an ophthalmologist. He could do a preliminary assessment of the disease's effects on my children's eyes.

Distrusting the System

I came home numb and terrified. I called Pat, my husband, desperately wishing he had come to the appointment with us. When you ask our children what they remember from that day and the following weeks, they reply, "The best Christmas ever! We got every toy we asked for!" We recall this period as a time of great fear and confusion as we delved into a morass of medical literature, trying to sort truth from fiction. Popular medical resources such as the Merck Manual described the condition in dire terms, including the possibility that our kids would die at age thirty. What most jarred us was the realization that the research-medical system was not a well-oiled machine. We began to understand that we could not expect accurate information or a course of treatment.

The only light in the season was our dermatologist, Lionel Bercovitch, who lived a few houses away and knew of our shock and sadness. He suggested we talk about the diagnosis and offered to meet with us at a neighbor's house, so that our children would not overhear our discussion. And so on Christmas Eve we learned about genes, recessive inheritance, pedigrees, and mutations. The doctor was frank about the limited understanding of the condition. A sense of foreboding began to overlay this already traumatic journey, which was starting to resonate with another experience — my brother's death.

My brother had died a year earlier of a lethal form of brain cancer, at age thirty-three, leaving behind a young wife and baby daughter. I accompanied my brother and his wife through his diagnosis, treatment, and death. All along the way, the doctors treating my brother at a major teaching hospital assured us that he would survive. After his death, I learned that his cancer is always lethal, but there were avenues we didn't explore because we trusted his doctors to lead us down the right paths.

From this tragedy we found that we needed to be active participants in health care decisions, even to the point of reading the peer-reviewed literature the next time around. We learned that helping loved ones through a health crisis was not like taking a number at the deli counter. If research on PXE wasn't being done, we couldn't just wait until they called our number — they might never get to it. So we spent the weeks following our children's diagnoses in medical school libraries, which aren't exactly lay-friendly environments. We faced steep learning curves. Pat was a design engineer for a construction company and I was a college chaplain; neither of us had any medical background. We copied every article we could find and brought them home to read, quickly learning that we also would have to invest in medical dictionaries; encyclopedias; and biology, genetics, and epidemiology textbooks. Pat poured all of his energy into understanding the science behind the research — his way of coping as a distraught dad. And every glance at the lesions on our kids' necks renewed our fear.

At the same time, our pediatrician discovered that a researcher at a major university nearby was conducting a research project to find the gene associated with PXE. She contacted the researcher, who came and took samples of our family's blood. It gave us such hope to think that someone was working on this obscure disease. We were thrilled to participate, even though the researcher provided no informed-consent process. A few days later another researcher called from another major institution and asked for blood samples. We told him to get some from the first researcher. How shocked we were to find that they wouldn't share and expected us to allow blood to be drawn from small children twice in one week. There was no central repository for the precious blood of people with this rare condition, whose numbers are 1 of every 25,000 Americans. We wondered if this was another indication of the inefficiency of the medical system.

Taking the Reins

Pat was relentless—learning the science as quickly as he could and bringing me along. Many nights he would read aloud passages from medical textbooks. We would bat the concepts back and forth, looking them up in medical dictionaries and encyclopedias. Sometimes we'd wake up in the morning to find we had fallen asleep with books and articles strewn around the bed. Sometimes we'd fall asleep in tears after viewing photos of sagging skin or reading about the deaths of young people from heart and gastrointestinal complications. We shielded the kids from this stuff as best we could.

As we waded through the literature, it became obvious that it did not present a clear picture and usually cited case studies that even we, with our limited knowledge, thought were extreme and unrepresentative of the condition. We also noticed that the few studies that included multiple patients contradicted one another. Pat's construction design work relied on project management and coordination; he couldn't understand why the same principles weren't applied to medical research. We began to scheme about what we would do if we were managing research on this disease. It seemed to us that not only did PXE need a central repository for blood and tissue, it also needed a large cohort of affected people to give researchers a comprehensive understanding of the condition's manifestations and progression.

We decided to meet with as many authors of PXE peer-reviewed literature as we could. Much to our surprise, everyone we contacted agreed to see us. Their perceptions about the condition ran the gamut, from one researcher who said, "PXE research is a rat hole—no one wants to do it, it isn't worth it," to some who were overly optimistic about the results of their efforts. We joined the only support group for the condition and encouraged its founding physician to let us help set up a central registry and sample repository. He was adamantly opposed to both, not wanting to share information with other researchers because he had given much of his professional career to studying PXE. We struggled for several months to work with him, but it became increasingly apparent that his agenda and ours shared little overlap. One long night, Pat and I sat at the dining room table over a bottle of wine and agonized over what we had learned. We could not wait for one researcher to make headway while this disease progressed in our children.

From our reading, Pat knew that just as he would coordinate the installation of plumbing and electricity in a building, so should the genetic studies, cell biology, animal models, and other aspects of the research progress on parallel tracks. Although it pained us greatly to do so (we had hoped that all affected people could work together), we started a new advocacy group for PXE. Pat's skills and mine complemented each other. As he laid the groundwork for the scientific endeavors of the foundation, I began to build the support structure that affected people would need.

We contacted the Washington, D.C.–based Genetic Alliance, the world's largest coalition of genetic advocacy groups. Its staff mentored us, introduced us to other lay leaders, and helped to focus our activities. With their help we were able to do a great deal in a short time. Gradually the new foundation, PXE International, took more and more of my time. I had been teaching part-time and stopped doing anything except establishing the foundation. We enlisted Dr. Bercovitch and met every few nights, so that within six months we had created the PXE International Blood and Tissue Bank, laid the groundwork for an epidemiological study, coordinated dozens of volunteer outreach efforts around the world (from those of a nurse in South Africa to a mom in Romania), and begun to build the PXE International Research Consortium. This process was not easy. Only a combination of the Internet, other support groups, and Dr. Bercovitch's help made all of this feasible. Our kids began to come to grips with PXE in their own way. Typical of children, they didn't take it too seriously and instead did things like naming a spider "pseudoxanthoma elasticum," proud to learn a Latin insect-naming technique!

Elizabeth and Ian have reacted to PXE in a remarkable way. They have skin lesions and the beginning signs of eye disease (although their vision is still fine). They feel most limited by a restriction on contact sports to protect their eyes. They have grown up aware that no one knows much about PXE's progression but also with ideas about how to fight for a different future. They have testified three times before the House Appropriations Subcommittee on Labor, Health and Human Services, and Education. At age eleven, Elizabeth recommended to the subcommittee that basic research be funded to benefit all conditions, not just hers. They both think that PXE has presented them with opportunities they never would have experienced. They believe that we will make a difference, so they don't worry too much.

Getting Researchers on the Same Page

Watching the disease progress in our children provides us with the incentive to work long hours and craft novel solutions. Our blood and tissue bank is one result of our efforts. The need for such a bank came to us from several different directions: My ever-practical husband knew that we needed a commodity to leverage if we were to have a place at the table; competing interests of researchers don't often allow widespread distribution of samples, which can slow research; and we knew that we would be able to offer affected people a centralized bank that would afford them something that they (and we) didn't have before—confidentiality and anonymity.

Despite everything we had been through, however, new lows were yet to come. Soon after we started the PXE International Blood and Tissue Bank, the researcher in whose lab we banked our samples actively tried to thwart access to the bank by other researchers. We were appalled, maybe naïvely so, that researchers would put their needs for publications, funding, promotions, and tenure ahead of the needs of people living with disease. We apparently experienced an extreme example of this, but we and other groups have encountered variations of it repeatedly. Fortunately, this problem was counterbalanced by interactions with other researchers here and abroad, with whom real collaboration occurred. One of these relationships led to a joint application for the patent on the gene associated with PXE—the first time lay people in an advocacy group have applied for the patent. We consider ourselves stewards of the gene and know that the real issues will be played out in its licensing.

Our foundation sits at the juncture of research, education for affected people, and information for clinicians. We coordinate the PXE International Research Consortium, in which nineteen labs work through us with one another. This allows labs to do what they do best—excellent science—while preserving the ability to publish their own discoveries. At the same time, the labs together determine the dates when information sharing will take place. This also lets PXE International see gaps in the plan and make sure that all research phases are simultaneously fast-tracked. For example, we saw that the most difficult aspect for labs was information and sample collection from affected people and their families. In an ever-tightening regulatory climate in which institutional review boards are scrutinizing all human-participant research, our organization provides a firewall between researchers and research participants. This setup protects patient confidentiality and encourages participants' involvement. It also allows us to recontact participants when necessary for research while at the same time protecting them. Participants can engage in an unrushed decision-making process with us, determining the risks and benefits of participating in the PXE International Blood and Tissue Bank, the epidemiological study that we sponsor, and other projects. They feel safe, knowing that we are all in the same boat—sharing the distress of living with PXE and searching for options.

Consumers as Catalysts

My work with PXE International has taught me that consumers can be central to the research endeavor. We can be a catalyzing force for translating research into the services we desperately need, such as treatments, technologies to alleviate suffering, and clinical methods of dealing with the conditions. I now serve as president of the Genetic Alliance. This role enables me to work with other groups so that we leverage each other's capacities to make a difference for our loved ones.

My family's experience also has showed me that we need strong protections for research participants but not overly onerous regulations that make it impossible for researchers to have access to patients. In the same way that we know that our nation's health care system needs overhauling, I am convinced that the research process in this country needs to undergo changes that will facilitate collaboration among labs and build large registries that allow discovery of the natural history and progression of disease.

We hope for a treatment that will slow down PXE and spare Elizabeth's and Ian's vision, but we know that the advances we seek are usually measured in generations, not lifetimes. For Pat, Elizabeth, Ian, and me, the journey has bonded us together in a profound way. Moreover, I know that when we shoulder our burdens with other advocacy groups, we will help to speed up research that will spare lives. It can't happen fast enough.

CHAPTER 5

TROUBLE IN THE RANKS

PROFESSIONAL PROBLEMS

⁓ Accountable but Powerless

Unable to deliver high-quality care, a nurse calls it quits, but not before blowing the whistle.

Barry Adams

Having grown up with both a mother and a cousin who were registered nurses, I was familiar with both the value and the inherent challenges of being a nurse. My own experience of being a patient who was hospitalized twice for open-heart surgery before the age of thirty also taught me the importance of competent nursing care. Yet nothing could have prepared me for my own sojourn in nursing.

The profession's sharpest dilemma crystallized for me during a 3–11 evening shift in 1996, after a nurse supervisor assigned nine patients to my care. One of them was a man with terminal cancer who required frequent increases in pain medication as his disease progressed. Following the institution's policy, which required a new prescription order for every increase in narcotic dose (rather than the more flexible range often allowed in care of the terminally ill), I phoned the ordering physician for the third afternoon in a row.

He informed me that he was very busy and I was not to call him again. Instead, he demanded that I get the order from his office helper. I attempted to explain that I, too, was very busy, being responsible for eight other very sick patients, and that I was required to follow hospital policy. I reminded him that it would be illegal for me to accept a medication order from an unlicensed assistant. Furious, he asked me to produce the law in writing. Embarrassed that I had never read the law, I agreed. I obtained a copy from the state nursing board; highlighted chapter 112, section 80B, which states that an RN can only receive medication orders from an "authorized" prescriber, and mailed it to him. (Only after I promised to mail the law did he provide the verbal prescription I needed.)

Volume 21, Number 1: 218–223. January/February 2002.

But after finding the law I needed, I kept reading. One particular line caught my attention: "Each individual licensed to practice nursing in the commonwealth shall be held directly accountable for the safety of nursing care he delivers. . ."

Hands Tied

At that moment I understood the contradiction that makes nurses flee a noble profession that should be a rewarding career. Although RNs are identified as the last safety net for the patient and are held to high standards of professional accountability, we have no authoritative voice in a health care system that often does not put patients' needs first.

I clearly recall a discussion at the family dinner table thirty years ago after my mother, who was a county public health nurse, was told by her employer not to discharge Medicare patients who, in fact, no longer required nursing care and thus no longer qualified for Medicare reimbursement. The object was to ensure ongoing revenue for the county public health department. Indignant, she protested. But she was immediately reminded by her supervisor of the price of rocking the boat: She might lose her job.

Most nurses in this country are "at-will" employees who can be fired without reason unless the firing involves discrimination or other violations of the law. We are expected to take commands from employers, even when the orders may not be in a patient's best interest, yet it is we who are held directly accountable for patient care and outcomes.

When I graduated in 1992 from a university-based nursing program, U.S. health care financing was in the middle of a dramatic upheaval. Viewed by hospitals largely as labor costs rather than as cost-effective, licensed care providers, nursing staffs were cut across the nation for the sake of other budgetary priorities. Predictions for the future of the nursing profession were bleak. I began my career wondering if a nursing education had been a poor investment. I decided that a variety of clinical experiences in different practice settings would be the best way to build my knowledge base and increase my marketability. Per diem employment in nursing was becoming the industry trend, so finding shift work to supplement my first job (which required day, evening, and night rotations) was not difficult. But no matter where I worked, it became obvious that an honors degree in nursing was meaningless when trying to provide high-quality care for nine, twelve, twenty-four, or forty sick patients.

Administering two rounds of numerous medications (intravenously, orally, or by injection) to a randomly assigned number of patients with complex medical and nursing needs was, more often than not, impossible in an eight-hour shift. Even the days when this risky drill was accomplished, everywhere I worked—two hospitals, one inpatient hospice, and several nursing homes and home care stints—nurses were voicing alarm that standard safety checks were becoming lost in the race against time. Commonsense error prevention measures, such as questioning the physician's medication orders and determining if the right drug and the right dose were being given via the right route at the right time to the right patient, were being overlooked. Furthermore, an increasing number of minimally trained, unlicensed patient care "technicians" were quickly becoming the hands-on care providers to a patient population growing ever sicker as hospital admissions and length-of-stay decreased.

Aggravating registered nurses' efforts to provide good care while being overworked was the need to comply with assorted institutional policies, individual insurer and HMO mandates, state and federal regulations, and an ever-increasing crush of paperwork. Ironically, the purpose of many of the forms was to document that patients were receiving the cost-effective, high-quality care that Medicare and private insurers expected. Which, of course, they were not. After only two years of working as a nurse, I decided that the profession was not for me, and I joined the growing ranks of nurses who were leaving clinical practice.

I accepted a position as a liaison for a community-based nursing HIV program. But, uninspired after a year away from patient contact, I decided to try again. I took a thirty-two-hour-a-week position on a newly opened subacute unit caring for patients with cancer, AIDS, and a plethora of medical and postsurgical conditions that required close nurse observation and medication monitoring.

Increased Medical Errors

Within months, as the hospital restructured to meet an anticipated financial crisis, the numbers of patients being cared for by nurses increased. As more nurses left, the ratios continued to climb to nine, twelve, and sixteen patients per nurse, even more on the night shift. To cover the gaps, nurses were working overtime and being floated to other units. During one particularly frenetic evening on an unfamiliar unit, I was given only a tape-recorded report and assigned ten patients with whom I was completely unfamiliar. I approached my supervisor and protested the deteriorating conditions. She supported my concerns but said that her hands were tied. The new staffing directives were coming from the hospital administration and nurse executives. I requested a meeting with the director of nursing. My supervisor told me, "There will be no meeting. She told me that if you want to keep your job, you will not do that [raise such concerns] again."

Potentially dangerous medication errors happened often during the months that followed. Insufficient nursing coverage resulted in more patient falls, poor wound care, and patients' going unmonitored or unexamined for hours. Despite minimal staffing, newly admitted patients continued to be sent to the floors. Patients' and families' complaints increased dramatically. Three patients were threatening to sue the hospital for lack of care and demanded transfer out of the facility. Adding to the growing alarm and indignation of the nursing staff was an employee newsletter in which the administration lauded, as an indicator of high-quality care within the facility, the recent three-year accreditation granted by the Joint Commission on Accreditation of Healthcare Organizations.

Blowing the Whistle

In 1996, bolstered by the language of the Massachusetts law on the accountability of nurses and my own observations of inadequate nurse-patient ratios, poor care, and medication errors, I sought out the director of the nursing department. "There are no unsafe work environments, only unsafe nursing practice," she said in response to my protests. A series of meetings that included the director of human resources followed. Within the month, despite an unblemished employment history and a personnel record that called me a "role model for nursing," I was issued a disciplinary action that accused me of having difficulty with problem solving and managing my time. When I refused to sign the disciplinary document, which would have signified my consent to the allegations and jeopardized my employment, I was fired for insubordination.

Together with another nurse who was disciplined one week later after reporting short staffing to the director of nursing, I sought out what seemed to be our only recourse. We jointly filed a complaint with the National Labor Relations Board (NLRB) for unfair labor practices. Another complaint from a third nurse, accused of patient neglect after raising similar red flags, followed. Six months after I was fired, a two-day trial was held in Boston. In November 1997 a federal judge for the NLRB ruled that I was illegally dismissed by the nurse executives in an attempt to silence and retaliate against me for expressing differences with management. I was ordered reinstated with back pay and the other nurses compensated for any lost wages due to the mandatory shift rotations that were punitively instituted after they, too, documented poor staffing. I declined reinstatement at the hospital; by then I was working as an IV infusion nurse for the Boston Visiting Nurses Association.

No Support from the Nursing Board

What followed was a game of duck and cover involving state regulatory agencies after the high-profile accidental overdose death of a hospital patient in the same month I was fired. The Massachusetts Department of Public Health, which I had previously contacted about conditions at my hospital, investigated the death. Its findings included two counts of patient neglect, two counts of lack of professional and technical services in the department of nursing, and several violations of administrative policies. But questions remained, such as how the facility achieved an accreditation by a federal regulatory agency amid a swell of nurses' concerns.

Of great importance to me and my fellow nurses was that the state nursing board violated Massachusetts law and its own regulations by ignoring my complaints of unprofessional and unethical conduct involving my hospital's nurse executives. The Massachusetts Board of Registration in Nursing is, in theory, supposed to investigate all nurses' complaints, whether they be about superiors or subordinates. Not only did the board refuse to do this, but in a wry turnabout, it later investigated me based on an "unprofessional conduct" charge against my nursing license by the hospital's director of nursing. After I hired an attorney, the charge was dropped.

This was the board that at about the same time held eighteen staff nurses at the Dana Farber Cancer Institute accountable for the widely publicized fatal chemotherapy overdose of a *Boston Globe* journalist. Accountability for this accident was complicated by the fact that the institute was restructuring at the time, no nurse was heading the nursing department, the drugs involved were experimental, and internal policies about the treatment protocol were not available to nurses. Yet the board refused to analyze the case in light of those special circumstances.

After I navigated my way through a labyrinth of several state offices, including that of the governor, the board of nursing requested that I meet with an executive committee to discuss my continuing concerns about the accountability of nurse managers. I was asked to bring materials or witnesses to assist them in the matter. I did so, but the board refused to hear from my witnesses or review the evidence, thus shirking its responsibility (state law defines the board's purpose as overseeing nursing practice and examining ethical and professional conduct).

More than four years of growing national attention, combined with a legal action charging the board of nursing with violation of Massachusetts law, forced the board to hold a full hearing. With observers packed into a small hearing room and a thousand pages of evidence before them, the Massachusetts Board of Registration in Nursing found "no evidence" of wrongdoing on the part of the hospital nurse executives. The board has a reputation among nurses nationwide as being unresponsive to patient care nurses who file complaints about nurse supervisors and protective of higher-ranking nurses. But I hear nurses around the country describe their own state nursing boards similarly, if not quite as severely. And there has been an exodus of nurses from the profession. I left in 1999, no longer able to see nursing as a viable career option.

Epilogue: After continued media attention following my case, the hospital's CEO and RN administrator resigned, the director of nursing left, and the hospital closed its subacute unit. The hospital has since created a new policy that seeks to protect employees from retaliation for "good-faith" reporting of concerns through internal procedures, including a toll-free "integrity help line" run by an outside firm. In May 2000 I attended the Massachusetts governor's public signing of a law that protects licensed health care workers from retaliation if they blow the whistle on unsafe conditions. Other states have similar legislation, but nurses across the country need the same protection. The cost of silence is too high, both for patients' health and for the health of the nursing profession.

⁓ Leaving Nursing

Cuts in hospital staffing have created conditions under which this dedicated nurse can no longer work.

RAY BINGHAM

I slammed down the receiver, planning to shatter it and rip the phone unit from the wall. I failed, but the loud crack startled my fellow nurses. Unaware of the reason for my outburst, they looked over in alarm. After all, I was usually the calm one. I stood by the wall, tense and trembling. To no one in particular, I said in a shaky voice, "She's our [unprintable] ECMO coordinator. She's got to [unprintable] know better."

Of the many frustrations and indignities I suffered in my eleven years as a neonatal nurse, that incident was not the first, or the last, or even the worst. But as I look back, I realize that it was the beginning of the end of my nursing career.

The year was 1995, a time filled with news reports of managed care, cost cutting, hospital reorganizations, and nurse layoffs. Our university hospital was not unaffected. One round of layoffs had already cost our unit several promising new nurses, and staffing cutbacks on our top-level neonatal intensive care unit (NICU) had trimmed each working shift to the bone.

High-Intensity Care

That Saturday morning when I arrived at work, I looked over the census and saw an overflowing unit with too few nurses. I was assigned to our sickest patient—a full-term, three-day-old infant named Dan. Baby Dan's condition had deteriorated so badly during the previous night that he had been placed on a heart-lung bypass machine treatment known as extracorporeal membrane oxygenation, or ECMO. A congenital bacterial infection invading his blood and lungs impaired his transition from a sheltered intrauterine exis-

Volume 21, Number 1: 211–218. January/February 2002.

tence to the postpartum world. In his brief, difficult life, Baby Dan had already suffered multiple ruptures of his pulmonary tissue, the result of high pressures required by a ventilator to push air into his diseased lungs. Two tubes, inserted between his ribs on either side, evacuated the air in his chest cavity. A third tube, exiting below his sternum, was needed to remove collected fluid in the sac around his heart before the fluid completely compressed his cardiac function.

The ECMO apparatus, used only as a last resort in dire cases, functionally replaced Dan's failing heart and lungs. The machine drained his blood from a small tube inserted into the jugular vein in his neck, passed it through plastic tubing to an artificial membrane lung for gas exchange, and returned it under pressure through a second tube into his aorta. Blood flowing outside the body involves a great risk of clotting, which we control by a continuous infusion of the blood thinner heparin into the ECMO circuit. However, too much thinning of the blood can lead to uncontrolled bleeding, and the fluid oozing from Dan's incision sites showed that his clotting was already severely impaired. I had to test his clotting every ten minutes to adjust the heparin infusion. In addition, he was on two other medication infusions to address his failing blood pressure, he required frequent transfusions of various blood products to supply clotting factors and to improve his pressure, he was receiving several antibiotics to try to combat the infection, and he required constant sedation to keep him from fighting us.

Only a year earlier any new ECMO patient, especially one as sick as Dan, would have been assigned two nurses—one trained as a specialist to monitor the ECMO circuit continuously, the other to provide constant patient assessment and manage other aspects of patient care. I was the only available ECMO specialist; working with me this shift was Amy, an experienced and savvy nurse who had helped to mentor me in NICU care. But recent staffing changes meant stretching our assignment to care for a second infant, Baby Jessie, a two-day-old infant born three and a half months before term.

Rolling Up Our Sleeves

Amy and I frowned at our assignment. Premature infants, susceptible to a variety of problems in the first weeks of their delicate lives, require careful attention. Pairing this fragile infant with a sick ECMO patient held great potential for disaster. We conferred with Fran, the charge nurse. She informed us that the unit was expecting several new admissions that morning, making all of the assignments tight. She already had called in every available nurse. This, she said, was the best she could do.

The primary responsibility of a nurse is to protect patients from harm. Although all three of us felt that this assignment was inappropriate, Amy and I agreed to take it. Working well together, we could handle almost anything—for twelve hours. Several other nurses, aware of our predicament, volunteered to help us whenever they could. With everyone on our nursing unit functioning as a team, I had confidence we and our small patients would survive the 7 a.m. to 7 p.m. shift.

But when I asked Fran who would be coming on for nights, she told me that the only two specialists scheduled for the next shift had just completed their ECMO orientation. I could not imagine handing this heavy and dangerous assignment to new orientees, so I planned to alert Marie—the nurse coordinator of our ECMO program who was to call later to check up—to the staffing problem.

Around midmorning I received her call in the back bay of the unit where we care for the ECMO patients. "How is it going?" Marie asked. I began to list Baby Dan's complications, intending to discuss the efforts Amy and I were making, the time and attention that our interventions required, and the difficulty we were having in properly monitoring a second patient, especially a sick and fragile premature infant. I barely got started before she interrupted me.

"But the ECMO kid is stable now, right?" she asked.

Incredulous, I sputtered briefly, then started to go over the list again, thinking she must have misunderstood the magnitude of the problems. She stopped me again. "Yes, but for the moment, he's okay, right?"

"Well, yeah, he's alive. With the pressors and transfusions, we finally got his pressure up a bit. And the oozing is starting to slow . . ."

"Good. I'll be out the rest of the day." She cut me off a third time and hung up.

"The Way Things Are"

Furious and incredulous, I could find release only by slamming down the phone and cursing. Amy came over. Still trembling, I told her about the conversation with Marie. She rolled her eyes. "That's the way things are now," she said, unfazed. "We need to get back to work." When others came and heard my story, they clicked their tongues or shook their heads, but they too were not surprised. I talked with the charge nurse. All she could do was change the ECMO pairing to give the night-shift team a more stable second infant. We had no time to dwell on the dangers of our present situation. We had sick babies to care for. I tried to forget Marie and refocus on the ECMO apparatus and the vital signs of the infant who was so dependent on my skill. We all got back to work.

But something inside me was missing; something had flamed out. I looked at the nurses around me. They had led me through the NICU maze and inspired me as a young nurse to enter the ECMO program and face the demands of caring for the sickest and most unstable of our patients. Their resignation to the unsafe conditions to which our once proud and caring unit had sunk—for the sake of saving a few dollars on staffing—alarmed me. Powerless to protect my patients, I began to wonder what I was doing as a nurse.

A Precarious Situation

Of the roughly 2.7 million registered nurses now in the United States, almost 80 percent are employed in nursing, and almost 60 percent of these work in hospitals. The numbers sound impressive, but a closer look reveals some ominous signs. The average age of the RN population is over forty-five, with only 19 percent under age thirty, and the growth rate of the nursing population has stagnated. Results of a survey published in the May/June 2001 issue of *Health Affairs* show that 43 percent of nurses in this country score in the "burnout" range on stress levels, 41 percent are dissatisfied with their present jobs, and 23 percent are planning to leave their jobs within a year. Nurses report widespread concerns with staffing, workload, ancillary services, administrative support, and safety—both the patients' and their own.

In the mid-1990s nurses were being laid off in droves as part of a risky, unproven, and ultimately unsuccessful attempt to slow increases in health care costs. Now, in the face of an aging population and an increasingly acute patient population requiring ever more complex treatment with ever more advanced technology, widespread reports indicate a shortage of practicing nurses to care for Americans' health.

Adequate Ratios Improve Patient Outcomes

A 1996 Institute of Medicine (IOM) study concluded that nurses contribute greatly to the quality of patient care, although the authors found insufficient evidence to support public policy on specific staffing ratios. A well-publicized 1999 IOM report showed that systematic breakdowns and errors in health care cause increases in patient morbidity and mortality, raising new concerns about nurse staffing and quality of care. A 2001 Department of Health and Human Services study found that higher RN-to-patient ratios resulted in lower rates of certain adverse outcomes.

To help address problems with quality of patient care and the workplace conditions that nurses face, many states have debated minimal staffing regulations. In 1999 California passed the first mandated nurse staffing laws. The state legislature is still collecting information and conducting public debate; final minimal staffing levels are expected to be in place by early 2002.

However, many professionals are concerned that hospital administrators will interpret legislated minimum staffing as the maximum ceiling with which they will be legally required to comply. This misrepresentation of the intent of the new law could lead to a decline in the number of nurses at the bedside.

Each day in intensive care is immediate and unique; each patient is on the cusp of life and death. Laws made in state capitals and based on generalized data and average ratings of patient acuity and nursing care cannot provide the answers. The judgment of educated, trained, and caring professionals cannot be legislated or averaged. Each day nurses take into their hands the lives of patients. Their own livelihoods, in the form of licenses to practice, depend on their ability to adequately care for the patients in their charge. The health care industry must learn to listen to those who provide the care. The health of the industry and of the patients within it depends on the nurses whose day-to-day, minute-to-minute contact has the most profound impact on individual health outcomes.

Over the course of our shift, as Amy and I started to rein in his many problems, Baby Dan slowly improved. Although he would remain on ECMO several more days to recuperate, he eventually overcame his infection and was soon discharged.

Baby Jessie was less fortunate. The very next day she developed a severe intestinal infection requiring prolonged antibiotic therapy and surgery to remove a diseased section of her bowel. Early signs of this infection might have been detected had the hospital not skimped on the cost of an extra nurse to monitor her more closely. The lack of sufficient nursing attention likely prolonged Jessie's hospital stay by months and added tens of thousands of dollars to her care. These costs well exceeded the "savings" accrued from not hiring an additional nurse.

Personal Toll

I did not fare so well myself. Only weeks after I worked with Baby Dan, Marie removed my name from the roster of ECMO specialists, to shave the extra costs involved in training part-time staff.

Soon after, in an effort to understand how the staffing cutbacks that compromised patient care contributed to our hospital's mission and enhanced our revenues, I attended a hospital-sponsored educational session on reorganization titled, ironically, "Delivering Exceptional Customer Care." I heard the business consultant, who was brought in by the hospital management for a multimillion-dollar initiative, tell a room full of nurses to avoid using the word "cancer." An oncology nurse asked, "What, then, do we say to a newly diagnosed patient?" "Try to say nothing," came this consultant's blunt and sincere reply. "The patient will associate the word with the hospital, and that's bad for repeat business."

Unable to keep silent any longer, I wrote a letter to my fellow nurses. "I recognize I am in an odd business. I want no repeat customers. Our patients and their families depend on us for clear, honest, caring communication. I will be glad to be laid off from this job, after someone has found an antidote for neonatal sepsis, a prevention for having to use ECMO, and a cure for prematurity. Until then, however, I am skilled at a difficult, demanding, and stressful job that not many people can hack. That is the profession of nursing. That is my value to this organization. And to my job I try to bring caring, gentleness, honesty, and humanity. Not 'customer service.' I feel polluted."

The next day our head nurse called me into her office and placed an official reprimand in my file.

The following month I stood at the front desk of our unit one last time. The unit was very busy; nurses were running to and fro, their faces drawn and weary. I looked over to the back bay, where I knew there was a very sick infant, a candidate to go on ECMO. In the forty minutes I watched, no nurse approached that bedside; they were too busy with other things. I struggled within myself. I wanted to run to the locker room; put on an old, familiar set of scrubs; and go to that baby to do everything possible to help him.

But I was powerless. I had come to the unit that day only to pick up phone numbers for job references. As a result of my reprimand, I had been laid off. At last, our nurse manager noticed me standing there. I told her someone needed to take care of that baby. She firmly requested that I leave.

I learned later that the baby in the back bay had died.

I don't know how many nurses like me have left the profession over the past decade. Although eventually I would return to nursing, by then it had become a job. It paid the bills, but it was no longer a calling or passion. Today I am no longer in bedside care. I work in an office, writing nursing research reports. I still feel about nursing as I always have, that it is an honorable and noble profession, affecting countless lives by providing a caring, honest, human touch in times of great distress. I love nursing. I just can't do it anymore.

⌒ Dolores

A young medical resident takes her own life, shining a harsh spotlight on the pressures of the current residency education system.

Daniel J. Derksen

Dolores used her purple Robbins pathology textbook to weigh down the gas pedal to commit suicide in her garage. It was fourteen years ago, but I vividly remember the phone conversation with the resident on call, the bearer of the very bad news. Dolores had died of carbon monoxide poisoning, he told me. Her death came as a shock to her husband, mother, friends, colleagues, and patients. She was a compassionate, caring person—shy but well liked by patients and staff. Dolores (not her real name) left behind no suicide note but many unanswered questions.

Volume 21, Number 5: 218–223. September/October 2002.

Dolores had been barely six months into her family practice residency training. As a new family practice faculty member, I wondered how we missed the warning signs. Suicide risk factors were certainly present—new employment, isolation from family, a stressful work environment, chronic sleep deprivation, considerable student loan debt and service obligation, and a spouse also in residency training. But thousands of residents year in and year out endure the same training and pressures without tragic outcomes. At the time—the situation has since eased somewhat—the stress and long hours of residency were a rite of passage, a boot camp that once completed assured privileged membership in the medical profession.

Wondering whether other residents in our institution's training programs shared Dolores's risk profile, I conducted a survey of all first-year residents. A high response rate (85 percent) showed that residents were keenly interested in the subject. The survey revealed that trainees working more than eighty hours a week were much more likely to have suicidal thoughts (22 percent) and be depressed (47 percent) than those working fewer than eighty hours (9 percent and 27 percent, respectively).

Hoping to prevent another tragedy, I presented the data at a hospital executive committee meeting a few months later. Several department chairs asked who would pick up the slack of patient duty if residents' work hours were reduced. The hospital CEO questioned the data's validity and commissioned the Arthur Andersen consulting firm to do another study—one that deleted annoying-to-management questions about depression and suicidal tendencies. Naïvely I had believed that Dolores's death and the compelling data would catalyze change. I had much to learn about hospital inertia and economic barriers to reform.

Overwhelming Strains

My interest in changing the physician training system was spawned by my own and my wife Krista's prolonged internship and residency experiences, Dolores's death, and my institution's resistance to reform. I didn't know Dolores well but had shared some of the same stresses of residency training. For example, when she was a fourth-year medical student, Dolores had not "matched" in family practice—meaning that through a computerized lottery process, an available residency position was not found for her specialty. She therefore followed her spouse to New Mexico and hoped for the best.

In our fourth year of medical school in 1984, Krista and I had unsuccessfully competed in the couples' match program. Unmatched, we scrambled to find programs that hadn't yet filled all of their training slots. Rather than residing in different states to pursue our preferred specialty residencies (hers in OB/GYN, mine in family practice), we chose to accept internal medicine internships at the same hospital.

To train in our desired specialties, in 1985 Krista and I went outside the computerized lottery system and obtained positions on our own. This move required a second internship. At that time, interns' work hours exceeded ninety per week; we were granted one day off a month and two weeks of vacation a year. Like Dolores and many other two-physician couples, we had large debts. We'd delayed purchase of a home and car and had to start paying off loans during residency. It was exhausting to work long hours and a struggle to scrape by, paycheck to paycheck. We didn't have a day off together for the first six months.

On a rare free evening together during our second internship, Krista shared some shocking news. On her way home from the hospital that day she had considered slamming the car at high speed into a tree. She was exhausted and depressed and felt that she was a bad mother to our then one-year-old daughter, Shannon.

We discussed the "microsleeps" that we experienced when driving home after thirty-six-hour shifts without sleep. We talked about how much longer it took us to read electrocardiograms and interpret fetal monitor strips when we were so sleep-deprived. It was like swimming in molasses.

One night on call, a nurse paged me to the ICU to replace a partially obstructed endotracheal tube in a patient on a ventilator. It was 2 a.m., and I had been soundly sleeping in the call room. Dutifully I tried to replace the old tube with a new one while the nurse manually oxygenated the patient and talked me through the procedure. But in my muddled state I could not thread a new tube over the metal guide. Fortunately, a second nurse's frantic page brought help from a senior resident, saving the patient an emergency tracheotomy.

A Different Approach Is Needed

I have witnessed disciplinary actions levied by residency programs against intoxicated or substance-abusing residents, presumably to prevent medical errors. Yet hospitals permit, even encourage, sleep deprivation and long shifts for residents, despite growing evidence that these also are harmful to both residents and patients. When investigating errors, hospitals do not usually collect data on physicians' or nurses' work hours and shift lengths. Yet it seems logical that overwork and sleep deprivation can easily contribute to medical error.

Recently, the Occupational Safety and Health Administration (OSHA), the American Medical Student Association, and the Committee of Interns and Residents advocated federal regulation of residents' work hours. The regulations limit these hours to eighty per week, provide at least one twenty-four-hour off-duty period each week, and curtail shifts to a maximum of twenty-four hours. (The Accreditation Council for Graduate Medical Education, or ACGME, instituted voluntary "work duty" guidelines in 1988, the year Dolores died.) In June 2002, Senator Jon Corzine (D-NJ) introduced legislation to make regulation of residents' work hours a condition of a hospital's Medicare participation. The legislation coincided with ACGME's report that recommended new limits on residents' duty hours—limits that were approved by ACGME's board and will take effect in July 2003.

These calls for change are needed. But despite my residency experience, I am ambivalent about some aspects of reform. The rigors of residency training build a solid foundation by combining critical medical knowledge with practical clinical experience. Following a seriously ill patient through a twenty-four- or thirty-six-hour course is a time-honored educational opportunity that would be lost with the proposed regulations. The intense training experience tests a resident's mettle, resolve, and intellect and teaches self-reliance and independent problem solving.

I remember at the beginning of a thirty-six-hour ICU shift admitting a sixty-year-old woman with congestive heart failure due to severe mitral valve disease. Her condition quickly deteriorated, and she was rushed to surgery, where her mitral valve was successfully replaced. To admit the patient, follow her through surgery, and leave the next evening knowing that we had saved her life was intensely educational and gratifying.

Another factor in my ambivalence about completely changing the status quo is residents' substantial contribution to physicians' workforce capacity. Decreasing residents' work hours could reduce access and services for poor and vulnerable populations served by this sector of the safety net.

But there is a price to pay for taking no action. When a resident commits suicide or when disturbing trends of increased substance abuse, suicide, marital discord, and depression are identified in the medical profession, reform is imperative—for the safety of both residents and patients.

A career in medicine is like a long-distance run—the pace must be measured and planned over a thirty- to fifty-year haul. Recent data suggest that during residency many physicians learn work habits that injure and impair them, result in premature death or retirement, or destroy marriages and other relationships at alarmingly high rates. Too much is crammed into residency training, while too little is invested in lifelong learning. Residency is not like staying up all night studying for a medical school exam. Doing that may have been enough to pass the exam, but the information is quickly forgotten. It may once have been possible to learn everything during residency training. But the exponential growth of medical knowledge and technology requires a radically different approach to physician education.

For example, physicians could supplement traditional lecture-based continuing medical education (CME) requirements with practical "mini-residencies" to enhance clinical skills and use new technologies. At our institution, field faculty precept medical students and residents, who, in turn, keep these rural educators informed about what is available online through the center's library. Some of these preceptors have learned clinical skills such as colposcopy through these mini-residencies or attended through the department's inpatient teaching services to keep their hospital skills sharp.

After surviving my own protracted residency training and that of my wife, and after training many residents and witnessing trainees' impairment and death, I still believe that there are ways to reform residency training without eliminating important teaching moments or reducing safety-net capacity.

What Works

As educators, we should better identify residents who are struggling and provide effective support, intervention, counseling, and mentoring. There are signs to watch for: poor evaluations, scarce attendance at resident meetings, disorganized medical records or oral presentations of patient cases, failure to answer pages, lengthy disappearances during the day, and concerns expressed by other residents. I remember one resident who exhibited several of these signs; it turned out that fellow residents suspected possible drug abuse. An intervention was arranged, and the resident received appropriate treatment.

We should consider adapting or codifying proposed regulations of resident work hours. While the old, voluntary ACGME guidelines were ineffective, the newly proposed regulations may be too prescriptive. For example, a thirty-six-hour shift without sleep might be allowed, as long as it is followed by an enforced rest period. Being in house in a nice call room while answering a few pages and sleeping for six or seven hours (a relaxed scenario that occurs with some specialties at certain nonbusy times of the year) is not the same as working all night delivering babies. Yet the proposed regulations would simply count duty hours and not allow flexibility across specialties.

The larger problem, of course, comes down to money. It will be difficult to wean our hospitals and training programs from a cheap, overworked resident workforce. Hospitals receive about $70,000 a year per resident from the federal government's Centers for Medicare and Medicaid Services. Residents' stipends and fringe benefits average $46,000. If residents' work hours shrink, calls will likely be made to extend residency training by a year, reduce stipends, or eliminate moonlighting by residents. But with the average debt among medical students exceeding $100,000, such measures will surely make things worse for the potential Doloreses among young residents and exacerbate the downward trend in medical school applications.

How to finance such reforms in the residency system is considered the biggest sticking point, but it need not be so. Perhaps Dolores would not have chosen to kill herself if she had received an average stipend of $37,380 for forty hours of work a week in a fifty-week year and if her overtime hours, defined as forty-one to a maximum of eighty a week, could have occurred either in the training program or by moonlighting. If her overtime had reflected fair market value for physician services ($50–$75 per hour), she would have had the resources to reduce her student loan obligations—easing some of her terrible stress. Such calibration would also reduce hospitals' temptation to exploit residents.

Doing Good for All

Incorporating moonlighting into a residency education program can be a win for all. As an upper-level family practice resident, I moonlighted on weekends by providing *locum tenens* (practice relief) coverage for a doctor in a community health center in Questa, New Mexico. That work provided a stress test that taught me what I was well trained for and what I was not. (As a result, I arranged elective rotations to enhance my electrocardiogram and suturing skills.) It also permitted me to earn enough to pay off our credit card debt.

In 1993 I helped to create, at the University of New Mexico School of Medicine, an academic *locum tenens* program emphasizing practice relief in rural and medically underserved primary care practices. These are mainly located in the twenty-nine New Mexico counties that are federally designated as having shortages of health professionals. In April 2002 the program had a record month, providing the equivalent of 300 days of primary care practice relief. Demand across the state, including in the Albuquerque area, calls for more than 500 days per month. Many community health centers, Indian Health Service clinics, public and private hospitals, urgent care centers, emergency departments, and private physicians are willing and able to pay fair market value for residents' time. Getting to know residents also gives these institutions a crack at recruiting them to their community after graduation. (Our *locum tenens* program is the nation's largest and oldest of its kind, but a few others exist, such as those at East Carolina University and the University of Kansas.)

Medical students, residents, and physicians in practice too often sacrifice a healthy balance between personal and professional activities. It is not altruistic to work more than eighty hours a week for our patients if by doing so we poorly manage them or sacrifice relationships with our own family and friends.

Dolores's journey in the medical profession ended prematurely and tragically. I hope that the latest calls for reform in the residency education system will chart a different course that allows residents to learn at a more rational and measured pace than current long work hours and sleep deprivation permit. The training regimen should be more balanced, more relevant to our lifelong vocation, and more respectful of students and resident trainees. Neither residents' lives nor those of their patients should be put at risk because physicians believe that they are immune to the effects of long work hours or sleep deprivation. They are not.

The stakes are huge. After all, any one of us or someone we love could be on the receiving end of a medical error committed by an overworked, stressed-out resident. And I never want to get another phone call about a resident's suicide.

⁓ Attending Death with Dignity

A nurse finds herself the center of controversy after effectively managing pain for a dying patient.

SHARON LaDUKE

Her name was Willie Dobisky. The widowed matriarch of a community-oriented family, she had been a wife, mother, Sunday school teacher, volunteer, and neighbor. For many years she and her husband had owned and operated the Surprise, a department store in our small rural town. As a child, I had been fascinated by the pneumatic tubes that whisked messages from one part of the large store to the other.

Willie had once been beautiful. Now in her eighties, her face reshaped by years of steroid use to control her emphysema, she was "dying by inches," as her son put it, and had been for months before landing in our hospital for the last time. In the emergency department (ED), lung failure had raised the carbon dioxide level in her blood so high that she did not have the mental capacity to make her own health care decisions. Anticipating this day, she had named her friend Mary, a retired nurse, as her health care agent. She had discussed her wishes with Mary, filled out an advance directive, and provided a copy to the hospital. But when Mary told the ED staff that Willie did not want to go on a ventilator and had completed paperwork to that end, the hospital could not locate the document. And Willie had neglected to give Mary a copy. Willie ended up on the ventilator.

Often when patients go on the ventilator, they can come off again and survive after the reversible elements of their illness are treated. But after a week it became clear that Willie's ailments were not reversible. Willie was a strong and proud woman whose quality of life had been poor for some time. She had always said that she did not want to live on a machine, and her loved ones supported her wishes. After multiple discussions among her health care

Volume 23, Number 3: 222–227. May/June 2004.

agent, her family, and the physician and nurses, the decision was made to have her breathing tube removed.

Willie's family probably thought she would die right away, but she did not. Her relief at being off the breathing machine, which was replaced by an oxygen mask, was soon followed by increasing dyspnea—a relentness, suffocating shortness of breath. Not like the kind you get from running up flights of stairs, but more like the panic you felt as a kid when your big brother held you underwater and you struggled to break free. Oxygen was being piped into Willie through a mask, but her lungs had failed, and she could not use the air. Twenty-plus years of nursing experience has taught me that dyspnea at the end of life is far more likely than pain.

Easing Suffering

Both Willie's family and her health care team had anticipated this problem, so the physician had written orders for analgesia and sedation. These drugs reduce breathing difficulties as well as the patient's awareness of them. Willie was to receive a continuous, pump-controlled intravenous drip of a morphine-like drug called Fentanyl and intermittent doses of Versed, a sedative drug. At first these orders were adequate. But as the hours passed and Willie began to tire from the effort of breathing, her dyspnea worsened. Despite the physician's promise to her three children that their mother would be kept comfortable, she was not.

By the time I took over Willie's care, she had been off the ventilator for a day. Every breath was now a struggle, and her gray face was contorted in a grimace. Her exhaustion and anxiety were preventing her and her frantic family from using the time left to prepare for their final parting. When I informed the physician that the present orders for Fentanyl and Versed were not controlling Willie's dyspnea, he increased the rate of the continuous infusion and wrote other orders that would give me the tools I needed to keep her comfortable. The new doses, however, were scary to me. Even though I knew that the only thing we could now do for Willie was to make her comfortable, I had never given anyone such big doses at such short intervals. I was, after all, a critical care nurse—skilled in preventing deterioration and restoring normal functioning in a clinical setting focused on life-sustaining therapy. I was trained for something entirely different from what was now needed.

However, I had recently been studying the care of the dying, particularly patients removed from the ventilator, so I knew that the new orders and plan of care were medically appropriate. I administered the medications as ordered. Willie stopped trying to push the oxygen mask away, sank back into the bed, relaxed her furrowed brow, and stopped gasping for breath. Family members then took turns holding her hand, telling her how much she meant to them, and saying goodbye. They recalled old memories and recited prayers. Because I was a longtime lead soprano in my church choir—the same church as Willie's, although I hadn't known her personally—the family asked me to sing "Amazing Grace" at her bedside, which I did. Within a few hours Willie died peacefully, her family full of gratitude.

Willie might have been at peace, but I wasn't. Despite my belief that the care that had been provided was appropriate, I had stepped outside my moral comfort zone into unknown territory. I had been driven by Willie's needs and those of her family but had given no thought to how I might feel about being the last person to medicate a dying patient. When Willie's suffering was over, the family home, and the documentation completed, I was alone with my thoughts and began to question myself. It is widely known and well documented that nurses and physicians can feel guilt after ordering or administering analgesics and sedatives to people who are dying. That's because these medications have a "double effect": As they ease or end the symptoms associated with dying, they can also cause vital signs to deteriorate—in essence, hastening death. Many clinicians have trouble on a moral level distinguishing between administering medications that might hasten death—an act that is required if the dying are to receive appropriate care—and giving drugs to hasten death, which is euthanasia.

So I was uncomfortable, and I'm not the kind of person who keeps things to myself. Over several days I told a few key people how I felt about this event, using the word *euthanasia* each time. My nurse colleague nodded sympathetically. My minister figured I was just grieving. A physician colleague (not the patient's doctor) said, "That's what we do. Forget about it." The nurse administrator, on the other hand, replied, "Euthanasia is against the law in this state."

Facing a Backlash

You'd think that last comment would have told me right then and there that I had to explain that my using the "E" word was emotional hyperbole. But I had a good working relationship with this administrator, and she had always been very supportive. I thought she would mull it over and that we would have more discussions not only about this patient but also about the hospital's end-of-life care generally. But she did not understand. She felt obligated to convey the discussion to the risk manager, and an investigation was launched. When I requested that the case be brought before the hospital's ethics committee, an administrator informed me that "euthanasia is not an ethical issue." Shocked into silence, I didn't have the wits about me to point out that the committee would help clarify that what had happened was not euthanasia.

One could argue that if I had kept my mouth shut in the first place, nothing would have happened. But ill-advised words cannot justify the subsequent actions of hospital officials. Although neither the internal nor the external peer review subsequently performed found fault with my care, the hospital reported the incident to the state department of health. The investigation then conducted by that department resulted in multiple citations against the hospital for failure to address the needs of the terminally ill and one against the physician, but none against me. Nevertheless, the hospital referred the matter to the state board of nursing and the county district attorney.

A few days after I met with the risk manager, the hospital placed me on administrative leave. I was paralyzed by fear and depression. I did my grocery shopping at 3 a.m. so that I wouldn't have to face anyone. But I also began to read everything I could get my hands on about end-of-life care. The more I read, the more I realized that I had done nothing wrong. In fact, I had done nearly everything right. My fighting spirit returned, assisted by a well-placed kick in the rear from my husband and the Dobisky family's outrage at the hospital's actions. I hired two very competent attorneys to represent me in the two different aspects of the case—criminal and professional (license-related). Not many nurses have the financial resources to do that; I was lucky.

After some six months of leave, the hospital offered me the opportunity to resign. Against my attorney's advice, I declined and was fired, as expected. What I didn't expect was that the hospital's lawyer would state in writing that I was fired for committing euthanasia or that the hospital's CEO would allegedly refer to me as "Nurse Kevorkian" at a public gathering. The disrespect and arrogance of these officials was galvanizing. After hiring a third lawyer, I filed two lawsuits against hospital leaders: one related to the termination of employment on a false premise, the other for slander and other alleged wrongdoings. The Dobisky family also filed suit, including among the defendants a nurse who had allegedly failed to provide adequate relief of discomfort for their mother. Now the hospital had one nurse facing criminal charges because she medicated a patient, and one facing a malpractice suit because he didn't.

Exoneration

With the filing of the civil suits, the story broke in the local papers. Shortly after that, the district attorney closed the investigation into Willie's death for lack of evidence. The threat of state troopers showing up at my house with handcuffs was over. Now I had to deal "only" with the professional disciplinary and civil aspects of this three-horned dilemma. I live in an at-will employment state, and in due time the courts found that without an employment contract I could be fired for any reason, even if the reason was false. That left me with the lawsuit for slander. As you might expect, this suit was not quickly resolved. The three years between the public disclosure of the accusation and the settlement of the lawsuit were not easy for me and my family, the Dobisky family, or the hospital and its employees. But I found support everywhere I went, from the administrative nurse at the nearby hospital that hired me as a supervisor in spite of everything, to nurse colleagues who lobbied elected representatives and other authorities on my behalf, to the state nurses association, which saw in my case the practice implications for all nurses who are caring for the dying. My church, the community, the local media, and even some independent-minded hospital board members also supported me.

The hospital did not fare as well. Headlines related to the case appeared with each new legal development. For two years it seemed that not a Sunday went by without at least one letter to the editor disparaging hospital leadership and its choice of "big city" legal representation. Board members confided that the hospital was losing its donor base. Pressure mounted to settle the case. Several developments finally made that possible. First, the state board of nursing did not find me guilty of professional misconduct. Second, two of the three administrators involved in my case had left the hospital, and the third had been reassigned. Third, at the suggestion of an influential attorney who came to my aid pro bono, I directly contacted the president of the hospital's board and suggested that we bypass our lawyers and see if we could negotiate a settlement. I had never been looking for anything more than re-employment and reimbursement of legal fees and lost wages, and the Dobisky family had pledged to drop their own lawsuit if mine was settled. So we were able to come to an agreement in short order.

I've been back at the hospital for almost six years now. It was a pleasure to hear a key physician refer to what happened as the darkest chapter in the hospital's history and to say that the only thing I did wrong was to be ten years ahead of everybody else. It was a long battle, one that most nurses would not have had the resources to fight. It was a battle I should not have had to engage in.

The War Continues

Unfortunately, the end-of-life care war is far from over. Much more has been done to educate providers in pain management since Willie's death in 1995. For instance, many nursing and medical colleges have integrated end-of-life care into their curricula. But despite a national push for such training, not all clinicians are competent in the management of the dying, know how to switch their focus from quantity to quality of life, or have the interpersonal skills to discuss such matters with patients and their families. Physicians underprescribe and nurses underadminister analgesics and sedatives, giving doses that make themselves, not the patient, comfortable. Evidence abounds in the health care literature that many doctors and nurses feel the same ambivalence I did. Yet end-of-life experts often are not brought in to assist with care until hours before death occurs, if at all. The dying are kept in the intensive care unit despite research-based evidence that even well-endowed university hospitals have been unable to ensure that patients in intensive care die comfortably. If I hadn't asserted myself about Willie's need for more aggressive pain management and been willing to personally provide it, she would have died exactly the kind of death that she and her family had sought to avoid, the kind that still takes place every day in hospitals across the country.

Government and hospital policies create risk for anyone prescribing and administering controlled substances. Legal systems tend to favor parties with levels of economic resources and expert legal representation typically not available to nurses. Ironically, while professional boards focus resources on the criminality of overprescribing, civil courts award damages to survivors for inadequately treated pain. "Angels of death"—nurses who have taken upon themselves to decide when patients should die—make headline news every few years, while angels of mercy struggle to carry out what the U.S. Supreme Court declared in 1997 to be the right of every citizen: effective palliative care, regardless of whether that care hastens death.

As Frank Dobisky, Willie's surviving son, told me, "Nurses should never have to be put in the position where they feel guilty for doing their job." Clearer, more consistent rules and regulations at state and institutional levels, together with stronger protections and support for physicians who order and nurses who administer end-of-life pain management, would help ensure that clinicians don't have to second-guess themselves when a patient like Willie asks for effective pain alleviation. Someday each and every one of us could be in Willie's position. As patients we will want our bedside nurses and physicians to have the support they need to best meet our needs for a comfortable and dignified death.

CHAPTER 6

DRUG RESISTANCE

BATTLING UNDUE INFLUENCE

A Matter of Influence   HOWARD BRODY

As Drug Marketing Pays Off, My Mother Pays Up
JANET R. GILSDORF

No Free Lunch   PAUL JUNG

∽ A Matter of Influence

Changing times call for changing policies on the presence of drug company reps in residency programs.

HOWARD BRODY

I was sitting in a room off the hospital cafeteria with a group of our family practice residents, waiting for teaching rounds to begin, when I asked them about the pledge taken by some doctors to "just say no" to drug reps by not accepting any gifts from them. Did the residents think that any of their peers would sign such a pledge? "Maybe half would," said one. "That's way too optimistic," replied another. A third resident explained that she would refuse to sign the pledge, not because of a desire to get freebies, but out of a conviction that she was educating herself before embarking on her career. How would she know how or whether to interact with drug reps later on if she did not gain some experience with them now?

About ten years ago I served on a committee in our department that decided that our residency site should make no effort to eliminate contact with drug reps or their gifts. We argued that part of residents' training was learning how to deal with the reps' blandishments in order to prepare them for their presence in later professional practices. I remain sympathetic to our resident's educational arguments.

Still, if our committee were voting today, I would advocate a policy that made our residency program—and indeed, the whole hospital—a "drug-rep-free zone." I would justify this draconian action by pointing to how much has changed in the past decade. The pharmaceutical industry has drastically, if incrementally and therefore often invisibly, upped the ante. Too much is now at stake.

Volume 21, Number 2: 232–234. March/April 2002.

High Stakes

Evidence is steadily mounting that we physicians are, in fact, influenced by the industry's largess. The proof does not by itself matter. What matters is how blind we are to the fact that we are being influenced. This lack of critical awareness seems to demand regulatory oversight. Today it is naïve to claim that each of us can make our own informed decisions about this matter. The likelihood is high that those among us who deny the loudest that we are influenced and who are most angered and insulted by this apparent reflection on our professional integrity are precisely the people who are most influenced and whose prescribing patterns are most deleterious to the well-being of patients.

Also, we must be aware of the growing scope of the problem as it extends its tentacles into every aspect of medicine. In the past I could entertain the impression that although I might get biased reports if I spoke with drug reps, I could always find the truth by consulting my professional publications. Today I have no such confidence. Even the most prestigious journals have published numerous papers by authors with serious, undisclosed conflicts of interest; and when a study reveals facts that are deemed unfriendly to the sales of a drug, the sponsoring company may use intimidation to prevent or delay publication of the results. Knowing how the few scientists who have dared to anger their company sponsors have been vilified, slapped with nuisance lawsuits, and had their research careers shattered, I conclude that a good many investigators whose studies revealed information unfavorable to a drug company quietly buried their data and never sought to publish at all.

The disparate pieces of this puzzle are interconnected. At first glance, whether our residents get to gobble down nice lunch sandwiches provided by the drug reps seems unrelated to whether a study's authors misrepresent their findings because of a financial conflict of interest. But why are residents so angry if a policy is proposed that will limit their free meals? Why is Harvard Medical School willing to look the other way with a policy that its faculty receive *only* $10,000 annually in consulting fees or $20,000 in stock?

Culture of Entitlement

What the residents and the Harvard faculty have in common is a culture of entitlement. Since the first day of medical school, we have been primed by the drug reps to believe that we had all of this coming. We work hard, we stay up long hours, we put up with a lot of grief and misery to become physicians. Moreover, at least during our long years of training, the people for whom we supposedly make all this effort—our patients—seldom express gratitude for what we do. Certainly, it is only small recompense that we get a few goodies now and then from friendly people who stroke our egos and make us feel desirable and important. The drug firms start the process of convincing us of our entitlement, but then we ourselves pick up the ball and run with it. The result is residents who think they are entitled to the tasty sandwiches, practitioners who feel entitled to dinner and drinks at the best steakhouse in town, and research scientists who think they deserve a lot more than their medical school salaries—and who, the school fears, will jump ship and go elsewhere if the school cracks down too hard on their perks. In an era of managed care, declining physician incomes, and ever-expanding hassles and paperwork, our sense of unfulfilled entitlement increases proportionately.

Regaining Integrity: A Better Lesson

Those of us in medical education cannot afford to let residents decide for themselves how to handle relationships with the pharmaceutical industry. Instead, we need to take firm action to reverse this culture of entitlement as thoroughly and rapidly as we can. Some of my colleagues think it is already too late, that the culture of greed, entitlement, and profit is here to stay. "Live with it," they advise. Moreover, a recent effort in Toronto to change the culture by banning contact with drug reps produced less than stellar results: Although residents trained at the program before the ban took effect today have about eleven contacts per month with drug reps, residents who trained after the ban have about nine per month—hardly a dramatic difference.

Yet I find myself unwilling to go down without a fight. Admittedly, once you have sold your soul, it can be a hard item to retrieve. But the medical profession today is not without financial resources. We physicians can afford to pay registration fees to attend unbiased continuing medical education (CME) programs rather than allowing for-profit firms that are closely affiliated with drug companies to organize our CME for us. We can afford to buy medications for ourselves and our families rather than dipping into the sample cupboard that (we tell ourselves) we keep only for the benefit of our indigent patients. If occasional nice lunches improve residency morale, surely the hospital and the medical staff, between them, can scrape together the funds. If our professional organizations now depend too heavily on donations from industry and our journals are held hostage to advertising, perhaps we can find ways to finance both through dues and subscriptions.

It's not clear what hurts more—that we have been so willing to bargain away our professional integrity, or that we have let it go for a bunch of ball-point pens and a few sandwiches and doughnuts. A strong effort to regain our integrity as a profession is a much better educational lesson for our students and residents than any number of "free" lunches and visits with drug reps.

～ As Drug Marketing Pays Off, My Mother Pays Up

A physician questions the value of a drug that may provide only marginal benefit—and why it was prescribed in the first place.

Janet R. Gilsdorf

M y mother, a North Dakota homemaker and wife of a retired businessman, is an octogenarian who suffers afflictions typical of the elderly: type II diabetes, degenerative osteoarthritis, and osteoporosis. This last problem is pronounced: Quite stooped, she is at least four inches shorter than she was in her youth. As a product of her generation, she doesn't ask questions of her physicians, nor does she seek health care information from her physician-daughter. To my utter surprise, she recently brought up a health matter, although in a roundabout way.

"Your sister says you refuse to get a bone density test," Mom chided me over the phone. I explained to her about the tamoxifen that I take in hopes of preventing a recurrence of my breast cancer—that it has the side benefit of reducing the loss of bone minerals naturally associated with aging and seems to reduce the risk of fractures. I figure that because I'm already taking

Volume 23, Number 1: 208–212. January/February 2004.

medicine that slows osteoporosis, the results of a bone mineral density exam won't lead me to do anything different from what I'm already doing.

"Well, I've never had a bone density test in my life," she said, a tinge of pride in her voice as if she'd won a contest of some sort, "but my doctor has me on something called Fosamax. It's supposed to work on my osteoporosis and, boy, is it expensive!"

I probed my mother for details. She explained that she takes a pill a week and buys four pills a month. "And that's out of my own pocket because Medicare doesn't pay for medicines at home." I know that she has no supplementary prescription drug insurance coverage, so she's paying the whole bill. "How much do you pay for the four pills?" I asked.

"Just a minute," she said. "I need to find the slip." I waited, listening to drawers opening and papers rustling in the background. "Here it is," she said a bit breathlessly: "$66.47."

"For four little pills?" I asked, incredulously.

"Yup."

Weighing a Drug's Cost-Benefit

As a pediatrician, I'm not intimately familiar with medicines prescribed mainly for older adults, so I had to look this stuff up. My usual first stop for such information is the *Physician's Desk Reference*, the legendary, massive, bright blue or red (the colors alternate yearly) PDR—a bible of drug information authorized by the Food and Drug Administration (FDA). I learned that Fosamax is the brand name for a drug whose real (generic) name is alendronate. It's no accident that the brand name easily floats off the tongue and readily sticks in one's memory while the generic name is harder to say and to remember. Typically, the company that sells a drug—Merck and Company, in this case—chooses the name, with FDA approval, hoping that we will bond to the selected moniker so that when the drug goes off patent in twenty years, consumers and physicians will continue to request and prescribe the only name we know (Fosamax). Every company on the planet seeks to replicate the Kimberly-Clark story in which tissues of all sorts, including the no-name ones from Costco, are commonly thought of as Kleenex.

Next I learned from the PDR that Fosamax, which is prescribed to slow the course of osteoporosis, lowers the body's levels of chemical markers associated with bone resorption (suggesting that it decreases bone loss) and significantly improves bone mineral density readings (suggesting that it strengthens bones). The kicker here is the word "significantly." As used in this context, it is a statistical term. It does not always indicate that the finding being discussed is biologically meaningful or medically important.

One of the oldest lessons of statistics is that you can find a "significant difference" in anything if you study enough subjects. In statistics, a significant difference is one that has a 95 percent probability of being real and a 5 percent probability of occurring from chance alone. For example, if you measure the pulse rates of thousands of healthy first graders, you might find that boys average seventy-five beats per minute and girls, seventy-four. A statistical analysis might show that this is a significant difference (with only a 5 percent probability of occurring by chance) and that first-grade boys have "significantly" higher pulse rates than girls. But in truth, a difference of one beat per minute has no practical meaning. In the real world of measuring pulse rates, these two values, seventy-five and seventy-four, are the same.

Back to my mother. I learned from the PDR that the bone mineral density for patients taking Fosamax improves between 6 and 10 percent after three years, and less than 1 percent thereafter. Improved bone mineral density measurements aren't what my mother wants; she wants to prevent fractures. Does Fosamax do that? According to the PDR, studies in older women who, like my mother, are already moderately stooped because of osteoporosis showed that after three years, 1.1 percent of those taking Fosamax had a hip fracture, compared with 2.2 percent of those taking the placebo.

So I said to her, "Mom, you have some choices here. Is it worth $66.47 a month to go from a 2 percent chance of a hip fracture to a 1 percent chance over the next three years?" Silence came from the other end of the phone. I continued, "That means with the Fosamax you would go from a 2-in-300 chance of a broken hip in the next year to a 1-in-300 chance. Is that worth the money?"

My mother has many fine qualities, but she was never a math whiz, so I had to explain this several times. Finally, I added, "You know, another way to deal with this is to prevent falling, which is how most fractures happen in the first place. About those throw rugs in the hallway . . ."

Efficacy and Value

What about the effectiveness of Fosamax, or any drug for that matter? The FDA is charged with assuring the American people that they aren't exposed to highly toxic medicines or subjected to medicinal hucksterism. Before licensing a drug, the agency requires the manufacturer to show proof that the drug is safe and is effective in what it says it can do. The drug safety tests are very stringent. Occasionally the FDA has to withdraw approval of a drug because with widespread use it is found to be less safe than originally thought. Examples include fenfluramine/phentermine (the so-called fen-phen obesity drug found to be associated with heart valve abnormalities), terfenadine (the antihistamine Seldane, associated with abnormal heart rhythm), and troglitazone (the diabetes drug Rezulin, associated with liver toxicity). This occurs rarely, however, and our drugs are remarkably safe.

The matter of efficacy is trickier. To be approved, drugs must be shown to be effective, but the degree of efficacy can vary dramatically and may be open to interpretation. What is valuable effectiveness to one person may be less valuable or ineffective to another. Related to effectiveness is the question of value—what you get for your buck. The rabies vaccine is considered highly effective in preventing rabies in people bitten by a rabid animal. How valuable it is in preventing rabies depends on the likelihood of being exposed to the virus. If you are imprisoned in a concrete-lined correctional facility for the next fifty years, this vaccine will have little value to you. If you are a veterinarian, the shot will be of great value because human rabies is uniformly fatal, although rare even among veterinarians.

So why did my mother's doctor prescribe Fosamax when the benefit for her might be modest and the cost so great? The answer is complex. One reason this drug and many others are widely prescribed is that they are heavily marketed. Drug companies spend billions of dollars to advertise drugs that are likely to have a large, sustained market because executives know that advertising works. This is especially the case for drugs targeting chronic conditions that affect large numbers of people. Just as magazine and television ads sell cars, hamburgers, pizza, and beer, they also are very good at selling medicines. The FDA has rules about advertising; the drug manufacturers often operate at the outer edges of those rules.

Physician Pressures

My mother didn't ask her physician about taking this drug. By nature, she'll just do what she's told. But many of her doctor's other patients, carefully schooled by ads, most likely did.

Other than advertising to the general public, drug companies also heavily target the physicians whose pens and prescription pads hold the key to company profits. Representatives from Merck and Company, maker of Fosamax, undoubtedly showered her doctor with company-prepared information on this drug, enthusiastically pointing out that it reduces hip fractures by 51 percent in elderly women who take it for three years. This relative improvement is technically true, but the absolute reduction is from 0.73 percent a year to 0.36 percent a year (calculated by taking the PDR-cited reduction—2 percent to 1 percent over three years—and dividing by three).

Even more important than advertising in physicians' decisions to prescribe treatments is the potential for litigation. What if my mother's doctor hadn't prescribed Fosamax for her, and she tripped over the hallway scatter rugs, took a tumble, and broke her hip? Hordes of lawyers lurk in the wings, eagerly awaiting the opportunity for such a lucrative tort case, ready to point out to the jury (with the drama of a Broadway production) that her fracture wouldn't have happened if her doctor had done his job. Again, my timid mother wouldn't initiate a lawsuit, but plenty of others would. Many Americans embrace the ethic, "If something bad happens, someone has to pay." Physicians and their malpractice insurance companies are viewed as open gold mines.

Why didn't my mother's doctor educate her about the small magnitude of the benefit she might expect from taking Fosamax, considering the amount of money she's paying? Because he simply doesn't have the forty-five minutes it took me to explain it to her. For an office visit, Medicare pays her doctor an amount that would buy ten minutes of his time. On top of everything else he needs to do in that slim time slot, he can't go through all the math and value calculations she needs in order to understand the issues and make an informed choice.

Is Merck and Company bad? No. Like any other large company, it is a business whose major goal is to turn a profit for its stockholders, and selling drugs is how it does that. It does what Nike, General Motors, and Kraft Foods do: advertise heavily and with a hefty dose of spin.

Does Fosamax offer any benefit in preventing bone fractures? Yes, but the extent of that benefit will be viewed differently by different people. Hip fractures can be very difficult for the elderly. The complications of being immobilized in bed while healing include blood clots (which could travel to the lungs, causing acute inability to breathe) and pneumonia. In addition, fractures might not heal well in older people. Is the benefit that my

Medicare-dependent mother can expect in light of the relatively low probability that she will fracture a hip worth the $66.47 a month she is paying out
of pocket? Only she can decide. Again, it's all about value—what she's willing to pay balanced against what she gets in return. Some people are willing
to spend $400 for a purse. My mother isn't one of them. It's easier for her to
do the subconscious calculations that tell her not to spend $400 for a purse
than those that might tell her not to spend $66.47 a month for one medica-
tion. The reason, of course, is that she is much more familiar with the value
of a purse than the value of a drug.

Like my mother, few Americans understand what they are getting for their
health care dollars. For many people, especially working Americans, such
decisions have been made for them by their benefits manager at work. And,
in health care as in everything else, Americans tend to want it all and to want
it now.

Is my mother's doctor bad? No. Like my mother and the rest of us, he is
a victim of a badly broken health care system. The appropriate fix for this
mess is as multidimensional as its causes and will require sacrifices and tough
decision making by many people. Meanwhile, my mother continues to fork
out $66.47 a month for the Fosamax, while the scatter rugs still litter her hall-
way floor.

～ No Free Lunch

*A young doctor's take on why residents' souls should matter more
than their stomachs.*

PAUL JUNG

A few months after settling into my internship four years ago, I found
a pack of M&M candies in my mailbox. Assuming that the chief residents were rewarding their charges with a little treat, I took the packet,
then noticed the sticker: "Compliments of Boehringer Ingelheim Pharma-

Volume 21, Number 2: 226–231. March/April 2002.

ceuticals, maker of Atrovent and Combivent." The same packets sat in most
of the other residents' boxes, and empty wrappers littered the corner trash
can. I immediately wrote a note to our program director, attached the
M&Ms, and placed both in his in-box. His secretary could tell that I wasn't
pleased.

Every year U.S. pharmaceutical companies spend an estimated $10,000
per physician on advertising. About half of the more than $11 million that
the industry annually invests in advertising goes toward equipping sales representatives with trinkets and toys that they dispense to physicians and residents at hospitals, clinics, and private practices. Debate rages over whether
such practices affect physicians' prescribing behavior. And some consumer
groups blame high drug prices on these marketing costs. Regardless of any
such link, the ethical question remains: Should physicians accept gifts—
large or small—from a company that may influence, or at least appear to influence, our medical decisions?

Gifts and Good Food

Pharmaceutical companies sponsored two or three free lunches a week
throughout my residency. These occurred during our noon educational conferences. Each buffet was arranged so that while standing in line for food,
residents had to pass by one or two drug reps, trained to talk up their drug
and reinforce their message with freebies such as pens, notepads, rubber
"stress" balls, stuffed animals, refrigerator magnets, and laminated index
cards with helpful dosage formulas. Americans bash HMOs on the grounds
that their decisions are based on money rather than medical need. How
would they feel if they knew that doctors' prescription decisions may hinge
on who pays for lunch? One study shows that 85 percent of medical students
feel it is improper for a politician to receive corporate gifts, yet only 46 percent believe that physicians should refrain from accepting handouts. We
physicians apparently hold politicians to higher standards than those for ourselves.

After reading my note, the residency program director issued a policy prohibiting any further gifts or ads in our mailboxes. He invited me to review
the policy on resident interactions with drug reps so that I could propose
changes to the program director's committee. My recommendation: No
more advertisements or gifts at our lunch conferences and no one-on-one

interactions between drug reps and hospital physicians. Instead, the reps could contribute to a fund to pay for lunches and receive recognition for doing so at the year-end graduation banquet.

I felt so strongly about this because the issue of undue influence is most critical during residency training, when young physicians' knowledge and decision-making skills are being nurtured. New medical developments are constantly emerging, to be sure, but residents should be hearing about them from faculty at educational conferences—not from drug reps at drug company-sponsored lunches.

Trying to Change Minds

At the next program director's meeting we discussed my proposal. Comparing noon conference sign-in sheets between days with free lunches and days without revealed no large differences in attendance. Hoping to sway opinion, I distributed copies of my annotated literature search, "There's No Such Thing as a Free Lunch." The research it cited provided scientific evidence of the effects of pharmaceutical gifts on physicians' prescribing behavior. For instance, literature shows that physicians who interact with drug reps favor the advertised drugs. This finding holds true both for direct financial gifts and for less direct interactions such as free meals and brief conversations with drug reps. Studies also indicate that residents who attend educational programs given by drug reps tend to overprescribe and misprescribe the advertised drug. Surveyed residents and physicians agree that such interactions compromise medical judgment yet insist that they personally are not affected. Despite this evidence, fellow residents on the committee were ambivalent about my proposal. So much for evidence-based practice.

At that meeting our program director gave us three options: the status quo, the "Jung plan," or the "high road," as he called it—a ban on all pharmaceutical interactions. As the discussion ended, he reached over and pulled a penlight out of my coat breast pocket. Expecting to see a pharmaceutical name on it, instead he found our hospital's logo. Relieved, he raised one eyebrow. "I didn't even know we made these penlights," he said. We ended the meeting with no final decision. He cautioned the resident representatives that no matter what our personal opinions, our first responsibility as committee members was to gauge the opinions and concerns of the house staff. Discussions with other residents revealed a common attitude: Residents were overworked and underpaid, so why not allow us a free lunch now and then? At one noon conference, a fellow resident pulled me aside to ask why I was trying to take away our free lunches. After a fairly heated exchange, he exclaimed, "You want us to buy our own pens?!"

Later I learned that the hospital's pharmaceutical and therapeutics committee had taken up the matter and decided to propose the high road—barring all pharmaceutical reps and their money from the hospital. We were told that this proposal obviated the need for a departmental policy. I let the committee's decision rain from above; it was guaranteed to be unpopular. As a chief resident put it, "There are good arguments on both sides, but no one wants to be known as the Grinch who took lunches away from the residents."

Back to Square One

Eventually the proposal went before the hospital's full graduate medical education (GME) committee. Almost everyone in that group opposed the ban. As the debate unfolded, one gastroenterologist remarked that a hospital-wide prohibition against house staff's interacting with drug reps would not adequately prepare us for the real world, where we would be bombarded with larger, potentially more corrupting gifts, such as drug company–sponsored research funds or plane tickets to sponsored conferences. The cheap toys we were given in residency were only the tip of the iceberg. In addition, if all lunch interactions were banned, residents would be flooded with offers for off-campus extracurricular dinners. These would not only be unsupervised but would provide free alcohol. Better instead to keep the interactions in house, with faculty supervision.

His solution was to require a faculty member to attend all conferences where drug reps were present. This would be easy to do; as a rule, many faculty attended educational conferences. The GME committee agreed that this was a good idea—akin to holding our hands as we crossed a busy street instead of prohibiting us from crossing at all. The definition of and conditions for supervision, however, were not made explicit. No one mentioned that pharmaceutical lunches with faculty "supervision" might convey tacit approval, even encouragement, to accept favors.

After this new default policy went into effect, faculty were indeed present at resident conferences. But their specialties did not coincide with the products being pushed, leaving them in a poor position to evaluate the information the drug reps were dispensing, let alone to screen it for residents. Rheumatologists appeared at lunches sponsored by Viagra, cardiologists at conferences sponsored by Cipro. And faculty never "supervised" the reps; maybe they didn't know it was their newly assigned duty to do so. They usually sat on the other side of the room, enjoying their subsidized lunch.

Practicing physicians are not immune to drug company goodies. In the home of an older well-to-do cardiologist, I once sighted an Evista clock on the living room wall and a box of Vioxx tissues in the bathroom. At a meeting I saw an endocrinologist wearing a watch displaying a Humulin logo with a small fork and knife as hour and minute hands. One would think that becoming a practicing physician with quadruple the income of a resident would curb the need for cheap baubles, but that's not what I have observed.

One infectious-disease faculty member pulled me aside and joked that instead of moonlighting, residents could simply rent the space on the back of their white coats for pharmaceutical ads. If athletes can have corporate logos on their jerseys and race cars, he said, laughing, why couldn't we do the same?

A Stopped Buck

I didn't think that the agreement to have faculty supervise drug-sponsored lunches went far enough, so I continued to try to set up a more effective policy. Without much support from my peers, I relied on our program director, a genial man who brought his own lunch to work every day. He was responsible for all final decisions about the residency program and often pointed to a placard on his desk that said, "The Buck Stops Here." I considered this a good sign, because he felt the same way I did about pharmaceutical marketing. However, a contentious issue required discussion in his committee and among the residents. Prohibiting drug lunches proved to be impossible when all but one resident opposed the idea.

Two years later, as a senior resident, I observed no change in the drug lunch situation. I was about to request a reconsideration of my original proposal, but more immediate concerns took over. The closing of several smaller hospitals in the city combined with a flu epidemic to swell our admission rates. Things got so bad that we were forced to board medicine patients on psychiatry and rehabilitation floors. House staff were swamped with work. My quest for an ethically clean residency training program, at first so clear, became muddied. In times like these, it was difficult to think that a free lunch here and there wasn't a small reward for our hard work. One final meeting with my program director near the end of my residency revealed an administration thrown headfirst into the health care crisis. I decided to let my point ride until things settled down, which they never did. I finished my residency with no significant change in the hospital's drug rep policy.

Feeding the Soul

One way to help physicians-in-training avoid the temptation of drug-sponsored lunches might be to have the hospital supply them instead. At $4 per meal for a class of thirty residents, an internal medicine residency program would spend less than $100,000 a year on providing free lunches every weekday. This is pocket change compared to a teaching hospital's total budget. Perhaps instead of trying to restore diminishing GME funding in Medicare, Congress could simply instruct the Centers for Medicare and Medicaid Services to provide free lunches to house staff nationwide.

Residency programs are charged with training and guiding this country's future physicians. These programs should provide an educational environment that sets us on a straight path toward appropriate medical care. Allowing pharmaceutical companies to pander to our hunger under the guise of exposing us to "real-world" situations is an excuse for convenient lunches. "An army runs on its stomach," my program director had said to me during my futile struggle to end drug company–sponsored lunches. In difficult times for public hospitals like the one in which I was trained, I can't deny this. But we must spend less time worrying about residents' stomachs and more time worrying about their souls.

CHAPTER 7

DISPARITY DILEMMAS

STORIES ON RACE AND ETHNICITY

Out of the Shadow   NEIL S. CALMAN

Subcutaneous Scars   VANESSA NORTHINGTON GAMBLE

No Come Nada   RICHARD S. GARCIA

Concordance   ALOK KHORANA

La Promotora   DARRYL M. WILLIAMS

Immigration Pediatrics   FITZHUGH MULLAN

∽ Out of the Shadow

A white inner-city doctor wrestles with racial prejudice.

NEIL S. CALMAN

Race prejudice . . . is a shadow over all of us, and the shadow is darkest over those who feel it least.

—Pearl S. Buck, 1943

I had been in practice in the Bronx for more than twenty years. Few surprises remained. After I'd been a family doctor for so much time in an area that had become synonymous with urban blight, the unusual had become usual. Treating patients with upper respiratory infections became a welcome reprieve from the challenges of helping single moms with acquired immunodeficiency syndrome (AIDS) to find a home for their children in preparation for their inevitable death, caring for patients with active tuberculosis, and dealing with an astounding number of middle-age men and women with hypertension, diabetes, and heart disease.

Nothing, however, prepared me for the day, three years ago, when James North sat quietly waiting to meet me, his new doctor. As was my custom, I moved from one exam room to the next with a fluidity that comes from years of practice, yet I was stopped in my tracks when Mr. North rose to his feet to greet me. His deep ebony, six-foot-three-inch frame dwarfed my pale, five-foot-three presence. The tremendous hands on his 260-pound body grabbed my own outstretched right hand and shook it, accompanied by a baritone "Good morning, Doc" that reverberated through the room. He reached around and closed the exam room's thick metal door behind us. I glanced at his face, trying to see through my initial discomfort, only to be greeted by my own face staring back at me from the silver, reflective sunglasses he wore beneath a baseball cap that covered his head and any hair that might have

Volume 19, Number 1: 170–174. January/February 2000.

been growing on it. His huge chest was tightly wrapped in a black T-shirt that, even in its largest version, couldn't stretch comfortably to encompass his pectoral girth.

At times like this, when some discomfort or distraction keeps me from thinking clearly, I am glad for the well-practiced scripts that have become part of my standard doctoring repertoire. "Good morning," I answered. "I'm Dr. Calman. What can I do for you today, Mr. North?"

He explained that he had come to see me because the cardiologist at the hospital had recommended that he get his follow-up care from me following his recent hospital discharge. He went on to tell me how he had suffered a severe heart attack that had left him barely able to walk a block without resting—this just one week after being discharged from the prison where he had spent more than a decade for manslaughter.

He recited a list of the medications he was taking, with the precision of a medical student seeking to impress his new attending physician. He also knew the names of all of the doctors who had taken care of him, including those of the physicians who were called in to consult during his hospital stay. My initial admiration for his facility in reciting this information was quickly replaced by my increasing intimidation by this man, whose size was clearly not his only outstanding feature.

It was during Mr. North's second visit that I became aware of the suffering he had endured in his fifty years of life. Not until I had completed the exam on his right eye did he save me the embarrassment of trying to see into his artistically matched left glass eye. His chest and abdomen were scarred from what I had come to recognize as multiple knife wounds. Now, left crippled by his recent heart attack, he was short of breath even at rest.

Despite his medical problems, Mr. North is taking charge of his health. He is now precisely managing his blood sugars, which in prison had been poorly controlled by oral hypoglycemics, with two types of insulin that he injects twice daily based on the blood sugar measurements he takes four times a day and writes in his notebook. His meticulous record keeping includes the exact date and time of every glucose test and every insulin injection.

Mr. North controls his congestive heart failure by monitoring his weight daily. His episodes of cardiac decompensation are always preceded by a few pounds of weight gain, and he now adjusts his diuretics accordingly. Al-

though his cardiac function (as determined by his symptoms, physical findings, and cardiac testing) is clearly borderline, he has been hospitalized only
once, for three days, for cardiac decompensation.

Breaking Through

Mr. North has become one of my favorite patients. This has happened not
merely because of his almost unnatural compliance with the interventions
I have recommended or because of the success I have had in keeping him
functioning optimally despite his cardiac condition. Rather, I think I like
him so much because he still intimidates me, and my continuing ability to
care for him allows me to feel special. I like him because I realize how hard
I have had to work all of my life to overcome the racist feelings that made
me fear him when we first met and that never allow me to act completely
naturally in his presence. I also love watching him interact with my staff because his commanding physical presence and intellect force them to deliver
a level of service I wish we could provide to all of our patients.

For those of us who have spent our medical lives in the inner city, fear is
always just out of sight. As health care workers we are rarely the victims of
violence, yet it is commonplace in the lives of those we care for. Mr. North's
sudden appearance in my exam room a few years ago made me realize how
vulnerable I feel at all times. Yet the most important lesson I learned was
how essential it is to recognize my fears and racial prejudices. This is a formidable challenge for a middle-class suburban boy, all grown up and practicing medicine in the inner city.

I have often contemplated whether, as a physician, I can rise above the
attitudes of the society in which I was born and live and the city in which I
practice. Can I learn to see through the faces of the people I treat and deliver to every one of them the highest quality care I have been trained to provide? Can I assist my patients in negotiating the racial prejudice that lines
the road between my office and the rest of the health care system?

I cannot provide Mr. North with all that New York's great health care institutions have to offer. He knows that. He has often tried to teach me that,
and just as often is amazed that I am unable to accept it. It comes up time
and time again when I send him for specialty consults, diagnostic tests, or
even prescription refills. The same considerations my family or I would re-

ceive are rarely given to him. The cardiology specialist who helped so much in planning a treatment regimen for his heart failure never thought of referring him to a heart transplant center for evaluation. It took three separate suggestions from me before a consultation was arranged. Mr. North has Medicaid. Although reimbursement for cardiac transplantation is possible, the reimbursement rates are so far beneath those of private payers, and organ availability is such a problem, that the likelihood of his receiving such a procedure is minute.

There is absolutely no doubt that Mr. North is treated differently than are my white, middle-class patients. The echocardiography lab where he had a scheduled appointment sent him home because he was ten minutes late, having had to stop every block to rest in the walk from his home to the hospital on a particularly windy day. The pharmacy refused to refill his insulin syringes without a written prescription even though he had been getting them at the same pharmacy for the past two years. I try to help in every way I can. Every time I send him to a new consultant, I call ahead with an introduction. I tell them how smart Mr. North is, how compliant he is with every aspect of his treatment, and how he knows so much about his medical condition and the medications he takes. I hope that my introduction will enable them to see my patient as I see him now, not as I saw him the first time we met. He needs that chance in order to get the medical care he requires and deserves.

Recognizing Our Biases

In my interactions with other health professionals I have come to believe that most of us have within us two types of prejudice. The first type is one we are aware of but that we have no ability or desire to change. We may recognize that the judgments we make are based on a person's race, sexual preference, age, disability, or other characteristic, but we do not acknowledge the invalidity of these prejudgments. We treat our biases as truth, perhaps admitting that they do not describe every person of a particular race, religion, or class, but believing that the generalizations these biases are born from are valid.

The second type of prejudice—and the place where I have been stuck most of my life—is recognizing my prejudices, realizing they are unjust, and consciously attempting to overcome them. This requires intentionally suppressing the fear and prejudice that rise up inside of me and deliberately making extra efforts to treat each person as an individual rather than as a member of a population group.

A hope I harbor, perhaps achievable only in a utopian dream, would be to remove the prejudices from our minds completely and to give people the right to show us who they are without our harboring preconceived notions about them. I know I have not achieved this, because I am still sometimes surprised to meet a new doctor on the hospital staff or a new member of our hospital's law firm and find out that he or she is black.

In Search of the Sun

Even personal victory over my own biases will not be sufficient to help Mr. North get the care he deserves. The New York State Department of Health looked at the use of cardiac specialty services among blacks in the state and found that, although they have the highest rate of hypertension and cardiovascular disease, the rate at which they receive sophisticated diagnostic testing (echocardiography, cardiac stress testing, and cardiac catheterization) is extremely low. Lower yet is the rate at which blacks receive sophisticated treatments such as angioplasty, bypass surgery, or cardiac transplantation. Studies abound showing that minorities receive fewer organ transplants and fewer technological interventions than do their Caucasian peers with identical conditions. Studies also show that for almost every major medical condition, the survival rate for blacks is considerably lower than it is for whites.

Society has a long way to go. Each Mr. North whom we health care providers let into our lives makes us more able to meet the next such patient without feeling the same prejudices. It has taken me much too long to get to this stage in my recognition of the views I grew up with in my white, middle-class, suburban hometown, and much too much effort to overcome them. Mandatory diversity training for all of our employees, a program that our institute began three years ago, has helped in palpable ways to improve the harmony among our multicultural staff and to increase each person's awareness of biases. The shadow of racial prejudice looms over us all. Training, coupled with constant vigilance, is needed to enable the sun to shine equally on all people.

∿ Subcutaneous Scars

A black physician shares what it feels like to be on the receiving end of racial prejudice, despite a successful career.

VANESSA NORTHINGTON GAMBLE

I was frightened as I drove slowly through the winter storm. Although I had lived in New England and the Midwest for almost fifteen years, I still did not feel comfortable driving in snow. On this day my journey was particularly treacherous—the roads had not yet been plowed, visibility was severely compromised, and night was falling. Furthermore, I was upset from events that had occurred earlier in the day.

A faculty member at a Midwestern university school of medicine, I had been invited by the dean to give a presentation about the status of minority faculty, residents, and students at the dean's retreat—a meeting that included school administrators and representatives from all departments. I jumped at the invitation. I had been appointed to the medical school's strategic planning committee and had been working to get the school to address issues of racial and ethnic diversity. This meeting, I thought, would give me an opportunity to press my case to an influential audience.

The morning of the event I set out early for the sixty-mile drive to the resort where the meeting was to be held. It was sunny, but the forecast called for snow. As I drove, I thought about what I wanted to say to my audience, most of whom I had never met. I decided that I wanted to let them know what it was like to be a person of color in medicine. I was one of the few black faculty members at the medical school, so minority students often came to my office to talk about their lives. They shared stories of triumph—making it through the first year, delivering a baby, getting into a residency program. They also shared stories of sadness—feeling isolated from their classmates; being mistaken (even by medical professionals) for janitors, maids, and dietary workers; being more intensely scrutinized than are their white classmates by security guards and attending physicians. Making my-self available to the students was time-consuming, and I often worried about the effects on my research productivity. But I felt an obligation to these students. If I turned them away, where would they go? Also, I felt that I was re-paying a debt; minority faculty had been there for me when I was in med-ical school.

At times my minority colleagues and I talked about the difficulties we faced at a predominantly white medical school in the Midwest. We talked about being asked to leave the doctors' eating area because we did not fit the picture of the typical physician, about a female patient screaming when a black man (her physician) had walked into her room. We realized that de-spite our credentials, achievements, and white jackets, our race would make it impossible for some people to see us as physicians. Yes, I thought, as I drove to the meeting, it was important for those at the dean's retreat to better com-prehend the experiences of people of color in medicine.

A Lone Voice

I walked to the podium and looked at my audience. It was overwhelmingly male and almost exclusively white, except for one black female adminis-trator. For fifteen minutes I discussed the experiences of minority faculty, residents, and students at my university and at other medical schools. Fol-lowing the style set by my grandmother, who was a storefront minister, I am usually a very emotional, dynamic speaker. But on this day I altered my style. I gave what I thought was a clinical, dispassionate presentation. I re-ported my observations about some of the obstacles that minorities in med-icine faced. I made my diagnosis: The medical school needed to create an environment that was more hospitable to people of color. I even suggested a few remedies: increase the number of faculty of color, augment the re-sources of the multicultural affairs office, add more multicultural topics to the curriculum.

I finished my talk and sat down amid polite applause. At my table sat the acting chair of one of the departments, who made the first comments on my presentation: "I talk to a lot of minority students, and I've not heard what we've heard here today. I doubt if it is an accurate depiction of what goes on here. I have a woman resident who will tell you differently."

I was taken aback by the hostility of his comments. I had not expected such a response. His words hurt. He was dismissing out of hand my experiences and those of other minority physicians. He was calling me a liar. He was saying that my words could not be trusted but that those of a white woman resident who was under his supervision could. He also was disrespecting my status as a senior faculty member. I was the first and only black woman tenured at the medical school, and I was very proud of that accomplishment. I wanted to cry, but I translated my hurt into anger. My voice rising, I retorted, "I will *not* be dismissed. Just because *you* have not heard the stories does not deny their existence."

The room went silent. My challenger went on to introduce the white resident, who said that despite some problems, being a woman resident was not difficult. "I just don't dwell on the problems," she said. Even more angrily I responded, "I will not be dismissed." Two female faculty members in the tense room tried to assist me. I don't remember their words because my emotions were so raw. I do remember that not one man attempted to help me. The dean stood up: "It's time to move on to the next topic."

I sat there for a couple of hours, feeling angry, vulnerable, and lonely. At lunch a few of my male colleagues came over to tell me that what I had to say was important. "Why didn't you speak up in the meeting?" I asked. They had no excuse to offer.

I decided not to stay for the afternoon session. As I walked to my car, the first flakes of snow began to fall. The only other black person who had been in the room tried to convince me to stay overnight because she knew that I was upset and that a storm was approaching. I thanked her but told her that I needed to get home, where I could feel safe. As I drove home, I tried to keep my mind on the road, but the day's events made concentration difficult.

I made it home without mishap, but as soon as I entered the house, I burst into tears. I cried because I was happy to have made it back without killing myself. I cried because I was in a place where I could feel vulnerable and secure. I cried because I was angry with my challenger and with myself. I was mad at him because he had been so hostile and rude. I was mad at myself because I feared that my response to him made me look like the stereotypical angry black woman—an impression that I did not want to leave on an audience who did not know me. I cried because I felt insecure in the profession that I had so long yearned to join. Although I grew up in a poor inner-city community in Philadelphia, I had decided at the age of six to become a physician. My family fought for, believed in, and nurtured my dream of becoming a doctor. I later learned that the pain associated with childhood dreams being rocked can be traumatic.

Other Times

The confrontation at the dean's retreat was not the first or the last time that an incident had wounded me professionally and personally. The first time occurred during medical school at the University of Pennsylvania. During my junior clerkship in internal medicine, wearing a lab coat and carrying a stethoscope, I walked into the room of an elderly white male patient who had been admitted for evaluation of high blood calcium. I introduced myself as a student doctor and proceeded to ask him questions about his medical history. Later, the white male intern came out of the patient's room and announced, laughingly, "You know what that guy asked me? 'Why didn't that girl clean up while she was in here?'" My being mistaken for a maid became a joke on the ward team, all of whom, except for me, were white and male.

The next morning on rounds the attending physician said, "Let's go see Vanessa fluff some pillows." I didn't find the episode humorous. I was angry and shaken. I was a good student at an Ivy League school and had begun to define myself as an aspiring physician, and I expected others to see me the same way. I might not be welcome in the medical fraternity, but they were going to have to let me in because I was qualified. This incident shook my self-confidence and threatened to undermine not only my professional identity but also my personal one. I had spent so much of my life in pursuit of becoming a doctor. Now it became clear to me that my race and sex would be an integral part of my professional identity. I would not just be a physician, but a black woman physician. I recall thinking that if I had been a white woman, the patient would have mistaken me for a nurse rather than a maid.

As I sat in my house crying, I thought of Helen O. Dickens, a black physician then on the medical school faculty at Penn. When I was in medical school, she often provided me with comfort and encouragement. I vividly remember one conversation in which I told her that at times I was made to feel inferior to my classmates and that I did not belong in medical school. She looked at me sternly and said, "The way I always figure it, for me to have gotten from where I started to where I am now, I had to be better than they were. You should start thinking that way." Dr. Dickens, whose father had been a slave, graduated from the University of Illinois Medical School in 1934; she was the only black woman in her graduating class of 175. Sixteen years later, in 1950, she became the first African-American woman admitted to the American College of Surgeons. Her personal integrity and professional achievements reminded me that black women have succeeded in medicine under circumstances much more difficult than the ones I faced.

Suffering in Silence

My talk at the dean's retreat did prompt the department chair who had challenged me to investigate my contentions. A week after our encounter he sent me a letter in which he tried to prove, once again, that I was wrong. He stated that he had looked at all of the student evaluations over a period of several years and had not found one in which a student had complained about racial discrimination. Of course not, I thought. When I was a medical student, I too suffered in silence, fearful of jeopardizing my fragile status. Although the episode that occurred during my medicine clerkship had angered me, I had said nothing to my colleagues. I had even joined in their joking. I was afraid to confront them and show my anger. I thought it was more important to get a good evaluation from the rotation. I did not want to get a reputation as a troublemaker; I wanted to get a good dean's letter for my residency applications.

The department chair's refusal to learn from my discussion and even consider that racial discrimination affected the lives of people of color in the medical profession did not surprise me. I have often found it difficult for physicians to discuss racism and its impact on their patients and colleagues. Many firmly believe that medicine is a profession that is immune from the values, mores, and prejudices of the wider society. As a black woman, I know otherwise. The chair was intent on maintaining the image of medicine as a value-neutral profession. My contentions punctured that image. The gulf between us was so wide that I decided not to answer his letter. I did not see the opportunity to respond as a proverbial teachable moment, only as a source of continued anger and frustration on my part.

Healing the Pain

The physician's letter made me realize that he had been right on one count: He and most other white physicians had not heard the stories about the experiences of people of color in the medical profession. Why? Because many of the stories are painful, and revealing one's pain involves an element of trust. As my grandmother used to say, "The three most important things that you own in this world are your name, your word, and your story. Be careful who you tell your story to." Besides, one often needs to bury pain in order to make it professionally, personally, and psychically.

Another reason why the physician had not heard these stories is that until very recently medical historians have virtually ignored black physicians' lives and contributions. At the time of the dean's retreat, I was struggling with what would be the subject of my next book. That confrontation persuaded me to write a book on the history of black female physicians, and thus I found a way to heal a painful experience. My hope is that my book will make it more difficult for these physicians' stories to be dismissed as easily as mine had been. (In tribute to my challenger, I have thought about entitling the book, We Will Not Be Dismissed.)

The history of my professional foremothers has provided me with a source of sustenance and reaffirmation. These women have had longstanding ties to the medical profession—the first black woman physician, Rebecca Lee, received her medical degree in 1864. They have also made valuable contributions to the profession and their communities. They and I rightfully belong in medicine. The history of black women physicians makes plain that I will face obstacles. Although I have had a very successful career, I will always bear the subcutaneous scars of racism and sexism. The stories of my professional ancestors reveal that their lives have contained not only trauma and scars but also strength and healing. Their lives and mine are testaments to the Negro spiritual "Balm in Gilead." Yes, there is a balm in Gilead to make the wounded whole.

⁓ No Come Nada

A Mexican-American pediatrician calls for nationwide backup in fighting childhood obesity among his patients.

Richard S. Garcia

"**N**o *come nada*," the Mexican mother of a two-year-old boy said to me at morning clinic, pointing to her toddler, who at thirty-eight pounds is far above the normal weight for his age. "He hasn't eaten anything in three days." The father of my next patient, a chubby three-year-old girl, worries that his daughter is too thin. "She doesn't eat enough." Another mother brings her four-month-old infant for an urgent exam because "she hasn't been eating lately." Finally, just before lunch my nurse warns me, "Dr. Garcia, you're not going to like going in that room." There, yet another heavy child waits whose mother complains, "No *come nada*."

The child "doesn't eat anything" is the literal translation of *no come nada*, but it is not what the Mexican mother of an obese toddler really means when she presents this complaint. Deciphering the code of Mexican culture in present-day California, I think the mother means that the child doesn't eat as much as Mama would like him to—that he doesn't eat as much as he did when he was a hungry, rapidly growing, normal infant.

I hear this chief medical complaint over and over again each day in the Los Angeles pediatric clinic where I treat mostly Hispanic children. It's usually not the ostensible reason for the clinic visit, but it emerges as the parent's most pressing concern. Each of these patients at morning clinic falls within the normal or higher range for weight; all are healthy. But the parents want me to stimulate their child's hunger. They want me to provide them with proof that their alarm about their child's "poor appetite" is valid.

Volume 23, Number 2: 215–219. March/April 2004.

The Clash Between Culture and Good Sense

I disappoint them each time, all the more so because I'm Mexican American; I should not only understand but should agree with their anxieties. My own mother shared the same beliefs about infant nutrition—fat babies are healthy babies—so I am intimately familiar with the push for more food. My mother wanted me to eat more, and still does even though I am now thirty-nine years old. She wonders why my daughter is so thin, why she "doesn't eat," why my wife and I don't force her to ingest food when she's not hungry. Ditto for my baby son. To want infants and toddlers to eat more is a Mexican cultural certainty.

But I don't agree with it. My chief complaint is that already-obese toddlers are eating too much. So I explain to each set of parents that babies with a fever, an ear infection, a simple cold, or just about any illness are not typically as hungry as when they are well. They are sort of like us adults in that way. I counsel one mother about proper infant and toddler nutrition and encourage appropriate meals, snacks, and exercise as my medical education and common sense dictate. In each exam room with a child who "doesn't eat anything," I try various strategies to convince the parents that their child doesn't need more food. By the end of a usual day, I don't know what else to say that might sway them. And whether or not I am successful with one mother, another anxious parent awaits in the next exam room, and the next. And more will be in tomorrow.

Few of these parents seem to understand that an obese infant is likely to become an obese toddler/obese child/obese teenager/obese adult. A 2002 surgeon general's report says that in that year there were almost twice as many overweight children and almost three times as many overweight adolescents as there were in 1980. More than 15 percent of six-to-nineteen-year-olds are at or above the ninety-fifth percentile for weight, according to the American Academy of Pediatrics. Five years ago the Centers for Disease Control and Prevention reported that nearly two-thirds of U.S. adults were overweight or obese; the problem has only grown since then. The girth of adulthood is nourished in infancy and prescribed by loving parents with good intentions. So I worry about what these parents' attitudes will mean for the future health of my young patients and their generation.

What can a Mexican-American pediatrician who disagrees with his culture's beliefs about feeding children do to treat childhood obesity, to help contain this exploding health problem? How can I practice "good" medicine, which includes advocating proper feeding based on accepted U.S. medical practices, if my recommendations directly conflict with the culture of my patients? American medicine, so far, has failed to manage the widening problem of childhood obesity, and I wonder how I can make a difference. Even if my advice is accepted and acted upon by a few individual parents, I know I cannot reach all the parents who harbor this chief complaint in neighborhoods and kitchens across America. Solving the public health problem of childhood obesity is a much larger goal than we pediatricians alone can achieve in our exam rooms—no matter how sincere and culturally competent we may be.

Formidable Family Forces

I believe that Hispanic parents don't want their children to become adults with the diabetes, heart disease, and hypertension that is associated with obesity. But the view that overweight babies are healthier babies is culturally embedded, reinforced by friends, grandparents, and history. These forces exercise far more influence over Hispanic parents than do pediatricians—even one of my background. The attitudes I encounter are solidly entrenched. Researchers writing in 2003 about Latina women's body image, weight, and food choices in the *Journal of Nutrition Education and Behavior* confirm what I see daily: Mexican women prefer "a thin figure for themselves but a plumper figure for their children." So it's nearly impossible for me to convince a mother that her child does not need more food. She leaves the clinic and goes home to a culture that disagrees with the young doctor.

Hispanics make up a growing portion of the U.S. population. In 2002 more than 13 percent of Americans were Hispanic and two-thirds of them came from Mexico, so obesity among Mexican-born families matters to the United States as a whole. But the problem doesn't rest within the Mexican or Hispanic family alone, nor is it due entirely to that culture. Purely American culprits include fast food, oversize restaurant portions, and children's increasingly sedentary lifestyles as they watch more television, play more video games, and sit before computers more often than any previous generation of U.S. children.

Certainly, government efforts to promote more healthful school cafeteria meals and more physical exercise for elementary and middle schoolers are a start. And congressional moves to combat childhood obesity are on the upswing. Last August the *Washington Post* reported 140 anti-obesity bills proposed by state legislators in 2003, double the number in the previous year. State lawmakers are pushing bills to restrict soda and candy sales in schools and increase physical education levels, to require fast-food outlets to list the nutritional content of the foods they sell, and to tax high-fat foods and movie tickets and use the revenue to carry out nutrition and exercise programs. And just as physicians advocate disease prevention such as vaccines and advice on how to prevent childhood accidents, we also push healthy eating styles and regular exercise to prevent obesity-related problems. Still, America is now home to the least healthy, most obese adolescents ever. Americans have evolved to a time when we eat in full absence of hunger. And what we eat is not good for us.

In a talk two years ago at a meeting of the National Medical Association, an organization that represents primarily African-American physicians, former Surgeon General David Satcher told the audience, "It's not about beauty; it's about health." He encouraged audience members to communicate this to their patients. He pushed more fruits, vegetables, and daily exercise. Dr. Satcher's recommendations would certainly lead us toward a healthier state. But how can his message be delivered to the people like those in my clinic who need to hear it? And, once the message is heard, what will convince them that he is right?

Ingrained Behavior

Laying out this argument as a medical warning to parents of toddlers can be interpreted as a personal affront. "I know how to feed my child," is the response I get when I inform parents that they might be overfeeding their child. Nor is the economic argument—the costs to families, employers, health insurance companies (and ultimately to healthy subscribers)—effective with my patients' parents. According to a paper in *Health Affairs* (Web Exclusive, 14 May 2003), this country spends $93 billion a year in health care costs related to treating conditions resulting from obesity or overweight. But telling my families that won't persuade them to feed their children less. Advice about health, diet, and exercise just isn't received well by the people in a position to do something to relieve the health care costs of obesity. I saw a woman on strike outside a Los Angeles grocery store the other day. She walked off her job to get more health care benefits while holding a picket sign in one hand and a cigarette in the other.

The issue I face as a physician fighting childhood obesity is the same as that of the rhetorician who looks at communication as a triad: speaker, speech, audience. Is the speaker the individual pediatrician in the exam room? What is my speech? If I argue that a thinner physique is a better physique, that not having diabetes in the future is superior to having diabetes, that being more productive and contributing to the world's economic machinery is better than eating butter, is the audience one family at a time? And what is the outcome? I can't help suspecting that with this approach alone, the country will get fatter while I plug away in my exam room.

Instead, it seems to me that a larger cultural shift is needed, akin to the movement against drunk driving, whose success in decreasing alcohol-related fatalities has taken several decades to achieve. (The proportion of alcohol-related fatalities to all traffic fatalities fell from 60 percent in 1982 to 41 percent in 2003, according to data on the MADD Web site.) That drop is likely the result of public education, enforcement, and new cultural attitudes about driving while drunk. Antismoking campaigns in this country have also been effective in reducing smoking. Such campaigns are needed to combat childhood obesity. Pediatricians and family practitioners are not able to keep up with the onslaught of human weight when treating patients one at a time.

Mountains Can Be Moved, Slowly

Change in cultural attitudes—both Mexican and American—toward feeding babies and toddlers and eating in general will be slow, if it occurs at all. But I have reason to hope. I have a thin daughter. My eight-month-old son is well within the normal weight curve for his age. And I have evidence in my own medical career that parents' cultural beliefs about medicine can change. I finished medical school in 1991. In those days my greatest daily battle was convincing parents that their child didn't need antibiotics for viral infections. Within the past year, while working at a clinic with affluent, white parents, I was confronted with a spectacular rhetorical problem: A mother who had been on the Internet, read parent magazines, and spoken with friends requested that I not prescribe antibiotics for her child because she feared he would develop resistance to them. I was at a rare and complete loss for words. I found myself fumbling to convince the mother to accept antibiotics for the bacterial infection I diagnosed. I assured her that I agreed with her concern about emerging antibiotic resistance but that this time antibiotics were warranted. The culture had changed in the other direction among this local group of parents.

The American problem of childhood obesity, which is so pronounced among my Hispanic patients, requires the full attention of private and public health care professionals and the agencies charged with education and health. It calls for a shift in the greater American culture itself.

Even yesterday, I saw a child and his parents in clinic. The Mexican-American mother was concerned that this boy, in the ninety-seventh percentile for weight but with two older brothers far above that, was "too thin because he's not like the other kids." I explained this essay to her and mentioned that I'd like to include her visit in my story. She smiled, agreed, and asked for a copy when it's published. She and her husband promised to go home and tell the grandparents what I'd said about how to properly feed their children. I wished them luck. And I promised to do my part. I imagine the day when, after mass education and a shift in cultural attitudes about feeding babies, I try to convince a Mexican-American mother that her child should eat a little more.

⁓ Concordance

How does a physician who is neither black nor white decide when race is a factor?

Alok A. Khorana

As I write this, my patient K.W. is dying in a private room on the sixth floor of the medical center. This is his second week in the hospital. K.W. is eighty-two, and, by all accounts, he has led a full life. The other identities he has possessed (amateur musician, Mets fan, preacher, fos-

Volume 24, Number 2: 511–515. March/April 2005.

ter parent, horror movie buff) have dropped away, and to my eyes at least, he is defined as the patriarch of a large and supportive family. There's always someone in the room with him when I do my rounds: usually a son, sometimes a granddaughter, and on weekends, his daughter.

K.W. suffers from metastatic rectal cancer, and I have been his sometime oncologist over the past six months. I say "sometime" because K.W. has never received chemotherapy for his disease. His cancer was metastatic when first diagnosed, and his initial surgery was complicated by a wound infection. This took several courses of antibiotics, and several weeks of nursing care provided by his foster son, to heal. During the past months, his family brought him in three or four times to discuss starting chemotherapy, but each time there were complicating circumstances, and we never got around to starting. In the meantime, his overall condition deteriorated, and he reported increasing tiredness. More and more he stayed at home, pushing himself only to make it to church each Sunday. Over the last few weeks prior to being admitted, he stayed mostly in bed, eating very little. When he was finally brought into the emergency room by his family some days ago, he was delirious, with high fever and a cough, and appeared to be dehydrated.

The team of admitting medical residents, mindful of my admonition to treat metastatic colorectal cancer as a chronic disease rather than a terminal state, did not discuss a Do-Not-Resuscitate (DNR) policy. Mindful as well of my other admonition not to emphasize race, the staff identified him on his admission note not as an "80-year-old African-American male" but simply as a "pleasant but cachectic 80-year-old gentleman." During his first few days in the hospital, we identified a pneumonia in his right lung, likely caused by aspiration. Worse, we found that his metastatic lesions had progressed significantly compared with the last scan performed just a few weeks ago. We administered intravenous fluids and antibiotics. K.W.'s condition improved, but only to an intermittently awake state. Most of the time he lay listlessly in bed, his eyes barely registering the images as his foster son flicked between BET and CNN on the overhead television. Over the next few days, I realized that it was highly unlikely that K.W. could improve much more, and I had misgivings about our ability to make him healthy enough to return home. Much as I hated to give up the idea of starting chemotherapy, I knew that my responsibility now lay in providing appropriate end-of-life comfort.

Making the Tough Decision

I had known the family for some months now, and over the past few visits had discussed the hospice option. I thought I had prepared them well for this final step in decision making for K.W. I arranged for a family meeting and was pleasantly surprised to see the entire family show up: sons, daughter, foster sons, granddaughter. I discussed, openly, how gravely ill K.W. was and how unlikely he was to improve enough to be able to receive chemotherapy. I recommended hospice. The family listened, asked questions, discussed the issues back and forth, agreed in principle, but asked for some time. Since K.W. was still on antibiotics, I felt it reasonable to give them another couple of days to decide.

This was a mistake, as I discovered over the next few days. As I had feared, K.W.'s condition worsened, and he lapsed into longer and longer periods of unconsciousness. I repeatedly tried to arrange for a follow-up family meeting. It took three missed appointments — the son showed up for one meeting and the daughter for the other two; both refused to make a decision without the other being present — before I realized that this family was having trouble making a decision. One of the nurses on the floor finally figured out what the problem was: The family was fine with transferring K.W. to the hospice program, but they were unable to commit to a DNR order. This was not surprising. I had heard anecdotally about the difficulties of approaching African-American patients and families regarding DNR orders, although I had previously taken care of several such patients without encountering this problem. A quick MEDLINE search led me to several studies documenting substantially lower rates of DNR orders in black patients. One large, community-wide study found that 18 percent of hospitalized white patients had DNR orders, compared with only 9 percent of blacks.

I have worked in the U.S. health care system now for less than a decade, but that has been time enough for me to become acquainted with the issues surrounding race and health care disparities in what is arguably the premier health care system in the world. I know, for instance, that African Americans and Hispanics constitute more than one-fourth of the U.S. population but just over 5 percent of physicians and less than 10 percent of nurses. In my chosen subspecialty, oncology, the numbers are even more stark. The American Association for Cancer Research identifies just about 2 percent of its members as African American. Patients from these ethnic minority groups are therefore far more likely to be treated by health care professionals from a different ethnic background: what researchers describe as a race-discordant physician-patient relationship.

I began to wonder if race discordance was important to my relationship with K.W.'s family. The Institute of Medicine (IOM) report *Unequal Treatment* (2002) described racial and ethnic disparities in health care in great detail. Although several factors are responsible for U.S. health disparities, the IOM report suggested that "bias, prejudice, and stereotyping on the part of healthcare providers may contribute to differences in care." Presumably, such factors would be less likely in a race-concordant physician-patient relationship. They might also affect decisions about advance directives. Indeed, in a study of AIDS patients, nonwhite patients with a nonwhite physician were four times as likely as those with a white physician to discuss resuscitation preferences. This might be related to better interpersonal communication in race-concordant physician-patient relationships. In a study of audiotaped physician-patient conversations, race-concordant visits were found to be slightly longer and led to higher patient satisfaction.

Neither Black nor White

As I read more, trying to gain some perspective, I discovered a big problem with the race-concordance literature: It didn't apply to my situation. I am neither black nor white. I am brown, but not Hispanic. I am also not alone. International (or "foreign") medical graduates (IMGs) account for one-quarter of this country's physicians, an increase of 160 percent since 1975. IMGs also account for more than one-quarter of current physicians-in-training. IMGs are important when discussing race concordance: One-fifth of physician IMGs and fully one-fourth of trainee IMGs are Indian, as am I. The next seven most prevalent nationalities are Filipino, Cuban, Pakistani, Iranian, Korean, Egyptian, and Chinese. The only predominantly Caucasian nationality on this top-ten list is German (just 2 percent or less of IMG physicians and trainees). IMGs are also of importance when discussing health disparities, because 40 percent of primary care programs depend on immigrant physicians, and two-thirds of IMG residents serve in hospitals providing a disproportionate amount of care to the poor. In other words, a black patient is far more likely to encounter a nonwhite IMG physician than a black physician. In certain Veterans Affairs and county hospitals, one is more likely to encounter a nonwhite IMG physician than even a white physician. Also, consider this: Given the disproportionate number of Indians in the physician workforce as compared to the general population, every physician-patient relationship that I (and other nonwhite, nonblack IMGs) participate in is, by definition, race-discordant.

I found little in the evidence-based literature to help me understand the issues facing K.W.'s family because much of the literature analyzing race concordance specifically excludes nonwhite, nonblack physicians and patients. There is grim irony in the fact that well-intentioned researchers—including IMGs themselves—scientifically probing issues of race and health care are treating as invisible an entire subset of providers and consumers.

This was remarkably frustrating for me. From my readings, it appeared that mistrust of a predominantly white health care system, based on historical precedent, and poor communication were the biggest stumbling blocks to DNR among African-American patients. Yet neither applied to me. I had been communicating well with the family for some months now, and I was confident that they trusted my medical judgment. Although indeed I was part of the medical system, my accent and skin color distanced me enough from historical acts of prejudice. Or, at least, so I thought. Was I wrong? Had I internalized the health care system's prejudices? Did this family perceive me to be making medical decisions based on K.W.'s skin color? Worse, were they right? Did they think of me as if I were, well, white?

A Simple Rearranging of Words

Finally, with K.W.'s condition worsening and my inability to guide his family to an appropriate end-of-life setting, I threw up my hands in despair and asked for help. The hospital where I work has recently developed a palliative care service, one of whose primary functions is to help families through difficult end-of-life decisions. Yesterday I called the palliative care team and explained the situation, expecting multiple family meetings before a satisfactory resolution. But only a day later, the white nurse practitioner on the palliative care service paged me to inform me that K.W. was now DNR and in comfort care and that she had already placed the orders in the chart.

I was shocked. How could she have helped the family transition to hospice so (seemingly) effortlessly, when I had been unable to do so for nearly two weeks now? "I called the son last night," she said. "I knew him from a previous admission, and he was fine discussing issues with me over the phone." But how did he make the decision? "Well, I helped him by not asking him to make the decision. I told him that his father was dying, that from my prior conversations with him I knew that his father wouldn't want to be put through ultimately futile aggressive cardiac and respiratory resuscitation. He agreed, but asked for more time to discuss things with his sister"—the same temporizing measure that he had used with me.

She continued, "I met with him earlier today. I asked if he had spoken with his sister the night before, and he had. But then he started to stammer and gazed at the floor. It hit me then. He couldn't bring himself to say it. So I gently said that we were going to recommend that his father be made DNR and have his primary team try and keep him comfortable, and I asked him if he had any objection to that, and, of course, he didn't." A simple rearranging of words, and an emotional burden is lifted from a family that is having a hard time dealing with a decision.

Had she used a similar approach for black patients and families before, I asked. "Oh, we use it for a lot of the families we see that are struggling with this, black or white," she replied. "If it's emotionally difficult for the family, I never make them sign the DNR; I just obtain verbal approval. They think that by signing they are deciding life and death, when you and I know the disease is doing that."

So there you have it. After all my hand-wringing and ruminating on race and race concordance, race was, in this case at least, a red herring. In trying so hard to not let this be about race, I had made it about race. For me, this revelation provided solace. There is no doubt in my mind that greater minority participation in the physician workforce is essential. But is moving toward greater physician-patient concordance a laudable goal? Race is, after all, a sociocultural construct. Should my sociocultural identity (immigrant, physician-scientist, Indian, bibliophile, Bollywood/Coldplay/Jay-Z buff) preclude me from taking care of patients like K.W., or L.F. (farmer, ex-veteran, white, Brooks and Dunn fan)? Should we start assigning our black patients to black physicians, immigrant patients to immigrant physicians, gay patients to gay physicians? Which sociocultural identity should be assigned priority when arranging for concordance? When F.G. (antique dealer, Caribbean American, gay) calls for an appointment, to which physician (black, immigrant, or gay) should our office staff assign her?

There are many, too many, problems of health disparities and discrimination in twenty-first-century America, but do we not close the doors to self-examination and self-improvement if we espouse concordance as a goal? I refuse to let go of my hope: Physicians are, if nothing else, educable. As health care providers and researchers, we are equally humanists and scientists; we betray both sets of principles if we are unable to move beyond our prejudices. We fail our craft if we cannot bring ourselves to look past the skin color or sexual orientation of a patient or, for that matter, the skin color or nationality of a physician. Zora Neale Hurston could have been speaking of an ill patient when she said:

> I was and am thoroughly sick of the subject [race]. My interest lies in what makes a man or woman do such-and-so, regardless of his color. It seemed to me that the human beings I met reacted pretty much the same to the same stimuli. Different idioms, yes. Circumstances and conditions having power to influence, yes. Inherent difference, no.

Postscript

K.W. lies upstairs. Tonight, or early tomorrow, he will die, or so the nurse taking care of him tells me. I have learned to listen to the nurses when they tell me such things. But he will die in comfort and with dignity. Dying is never easy, but it can be made easier; and for K.W., we have made it easier. And he will die surrounded by family—a family relieved, semantically but also emotionally, of the burden of a difficult decision. There is solace in all of this too, is there not?

∿ La Promotora

Linking disenfranchised residents along the border to the U.S. health care system.

Darryl M. Williams

O n the hot June day I arrived, Lorenza was sitting in her makeshift office in the double-wide mobile home that served as the clinic. Her government-issue metal desk was pushed against the wall next to a filing cabinet whose handles were loose and hanging down. She had a map of the *colonias* thumbtacked to the wall and a stack of appointments lined up on the seat of a folding chair. She asked if I would like to help her hand out fliers to the community, and I said sure.

Lorenza was the *promotora de salud* (health promoter) for the San Elizario clinic in far eastern El Paso County, Texas, near the Mexican border. The clinic served a group of *colonias* inhabited by some 10,000 people. *Colonias* are unincorporated developments without public services — no water, sewage, or electricity. This cluster of them was created about twenty years ago when land developers broke up the fertile bottomland of the Rio Grande into quarter-acre parcels. The little plots were sold to families from the barrios of downtown El Paso who were anxious to make a better life for their children in the country. I was there to work in some of Texas Tech's outreach clinics, created to provide health care to *colonia* residents through shared teaching with the local nursing school at the University of Texas at El Paso.

Fitting In

My academic career had been like many others, progressing from clinical training to research lab to administration. I had been away from patient care for some time and was looking forward to seeing patients again and to teach-

Volume 20, Number 3: 212–218. May/June 2001.

ing Texas Tech medical students, residents, and nurses training in the *colonias'* clinics. I was a bit nervous about the endeavor because my clinical skills were a little rusty after so many years of paper pushing, and my Spanish abilities were nil.

Lorenza's job was to know who was sick, who was pregnant, and who was not taking prescribed medications so that she could visit them at home and make arrangements for care. In the mornings she helped in the clinic by taking vital signs and translating for patients. In the afternoons she made her rounds in the community. She also offered classes to women in basic homemaking skills, parenting, first aid, and sanitation. She had studied these topics in a clinic-provided course for community volunteers. The class had been designed by a social worker who had patterned the curriculum on one used in her native Mexico for volunteers. Unlike in Mexico, in this American clinic the *promotoras* would be paid employees.

As we loaded into my car with the fliers, she explained that if *colonia* residents missed a payment to the developer who had provided them loans, he would foreclose on the land and sell it out from under them. The families who bought these plots worked hard to make them livable, building shallow wells and privies. Their lack of public health awareness led to endemic diseases such as hepatitis A. El Paso County contains more than a hundred *colonias*, many of them in the desert. The state of Texas has thousands of *colonias*, which some 300,000 people call home. Similar communities exist in the border states of California, Arizona, and New Mexico.

The Local Scene

Some of the houses in the *colonias* were made from wooden shipping pallets and cardboard boxes; others had cinder-block additions and artistic brickwork. A tall fence and a herd of goats surrounded one house. A huge storage yard for rented portable toilets stood in the middle of the community. A wide canal that had once served as a cesspool had been drained and turned into a children's playground. As I went door to door with Lorenza, we handed out fliers about parenting classes to a few interested housewives. At the last street, a few yards from the Rio Grande and the Mexican border, some young men stood next to a car with out-of-state tags, fixing binoculars on the sagebrush across the river. "Drug dealers waiting for a shipment," pronounced Lorenza.

Learning from Lorenza

That first day marked the start of a several-year collaboration with Lorenza to get patients into the clinic, explain treatment plans, and follow up on care. Through her I learned much about how to begin handling the public health challenges in these communities.

For example, in the medical center we are often too quick to label patients as "noncompliant" and move on to the next case. When a patient in the clinic wasn't taking medication we had prescribed, Lorenza would investigate, often discovering that the family had no money to buy the drug. She engaged in various counterattacks, including trying to get the patient on Medicaid, applying for indigent care at the county hospital, setting up a deal with the local pharmacy, or even buying the medications with her own money.

We worried about nutrition and diabetes in the *colonias,* and Lorenza started a nutrition class that involved cooking lessons and trips to the grocery store. She found ways to help families get food by brokering loans with the small food shops or getting neighbors to contribute groceries. We worried about gang activity, and Lorenza confronted a group of "taggers"—adolescent boys who sprayed their gang's initials on property to mark their territory—who had splashed graffiti on a historical building. The graffiti stopped. We worried about teenage pregnancy, and Lorenza created a support group for teenage girls. When a child came to the clinic with burns from a home fire, Lorenza visited his home, a windowless trailer. This inspired the entire clinic staff to pitch in for windows, blankets, a safe heater, and toys.

Equally important for Anglo clinic staff and students alike, Lorenza provided a window into the local culture. As part of our curriculum we invited presentations focusing on Mexican culture. One time she filled in for a local *curandera*—a traditional faith healer—who had cancelled a session about common folk remedies and curing rituals. Lorenza arrived for the session looking like a different person. She had pulled her long black hair into a single braid that hung down her back and heavily shadowed her eyes. She wore dangling hoop earrings with blue stones and a long, intricately patterned, handwoven skirt. Under her arms she carried a striped blanket enclosing some candles and an assortment of strange bottles. She arranged the blanket over one of the tables in the clinic conference room, spread out the bottles, and lit the candles. She explained how the contents of the bottles could be used for various ailments and then performed a *limpia* — a cleansing rite for someone with a treatment-resistant fever or illness.

Lorenza spoke in a low voice while passing a hen's egg over me — her volunteer, pressed into service when the students held back. She swirled the egg through the air and spoke in Spanish in semi-intelligible prayer. After several minutes she looked upward, spread her arms, and became silent. She reached down, cracked the egg into a small bowl, and placed it on the floor beneath me. Later Lorenza told me she had dressed that way to remember from where she has come. She believes in modern medicine but is a religious person with faith in the power of herbs and traditional remedies.

The Making of a *Promotora*

I learned that Lorenza had been a single mother, raising two children in a one-room adobe house with a dirt floor. Her husband was an abusive drunk, and she divorced him. At that point she had never worked outside the home and had little education or skills beyond those gleaned from migrant farm worker camps in California and Oregon.

Lorenza's first job was in an El Paso garment factory. Sewing an endless supply of buttons on an endless supply of denim pants wasn't much of a challenge, but it was a start. Soon she was a supervisor, traveling to other factories to train new workers and new supervisors. Over time she felt she could not continue because being a supervisor required her to choose sides, often against her friends in the production line. She began to help neighbors, speak out about nutrition in the schools, and work for community cleanup efforts — activities that led to her training as a *promotora* and to her clinic job. From there she was elected to the school board and, after a bout with cancer, joined the board of the El Paso chapter of the American Cancer Society.

Today Lorenza is a member of the inaugural class for *promotoras* at El Paso Community College. She is also working for a project in which she prepares other *promotoras* to teach mothers and grandmothers about infant care.

In my current clinic work along the border I continue to observe firsthand the effectiveness of Lorenza and other *promotoras* in helping their wrenchingly poor communities. Rooted in the culture of the *colonias* and trusted by their residents, *promotoras* know about family situations that need attention and that influence the success of a patient's management. Recently they have demonstrated that they can successfully recruit enrollment in the State Children's Health Insurance Program (SCHIP) when more conventional efforts have failed. Immigrant populations are leery of SCHIP because they suspect that it may be used to block citizenship applications for a family member. They are intimidated by the program's application forms and unclear about SCHIP's benefits. *Promotoras* go to people's homes to explain how the program works, a method that has been more effective in expanding enrollment among immigrant groups than high-tech, media-based campaigns have been.

Lorenza understood the potential for *promotoras* to become an important force in health care delivery along the border even more clearly than I did. When the opportunity arose for her to organize and speak up for *promotoras*, she grabbed it. In 1996 Texas Tech's Office of Border Health became a subcontractor for the Border Vision Fronteriza project of the University of Arizona, funded by the federal Health Resources and Services Administration. We were tasked with developing a curriculum for a train-the-trainer program for *promotoras*, field testing the program, and enlisting women to participate. Lorenza joined our office staff and played a lead role in implementing the program. She saw that what was missing was recognition of the value of *promotoras* and a general agreement that they should be paid for their work. (Some clinics—not ours—thought that women in the *colonias* should be willing to volunteer a forty-hour week for the sake of their community!)

As we sat in the clinic over many a lunch of *burritos, gorditas,* or *flautas* bought from local vendors, Lorenza proposed to me and others that there should be a standardized educational process for *promotoras* that would permit certification and, in turn, mobility. With mobility would come a broad job market and an opportunity for impoverished women who had never worked outside of the home to make a living and help to support their families.

Replicating a Good Thing

These ideas have caught on. Clinics and hospitals all along the border are hiring *promotoras*. Many communities in other parts of Texas and in other border states are establishing training programs and organizing groups of community health workers. Interested visitors from all over the country have come to the four Kellogg Community Partnership clinics in the past few years. Parallel to these rural initiatives, national interest is growing in using community-based workers to help address the health and social problems of ethnic communities in our inner cities.

Detractors might say that the role of these individuals has not been convincingly demonstrated in measurable outcomes. I need only recall the scores of patients I have seen who have turned the corner in trying to take control of their illnesses after an encounter with a *promotora*. To many immigrants who live along the U.S.–Mexico border, effective, aggressive *promotoras* are the sole link to the health care system. Beyond the humanitarian reasons to engage *promotoras* in improving health care for border residents, national interests argue for doing so. The border is a fragile buffer zone dividing the rest of the country from a host of infectious diseases and other health issues faced by impoverished immigrants. Bolstering the work of the *promotoras* along the border could well help to protect the health of us all.

Bringing *Promotoras* into the System

Three tasks lie ahead of us before we can enlist *promotoras* as permanent members of the health care team. We must make sure that *promotoras* have been adequately trained to assume the significant responsibilities they are often given, that the training programs used are of demonstrably high and consistent quality, and that we find the means to ensure that *promotoras* receive a living wage and are not expected to work only as volunteers.

Help may be on the way. During its 1999 session the Texas state legislature charged the state's department of health with establishing a statewide advisory committee to examine the role of the *promotora* in health care delivery. This committee is defining a core curriculum for *promotoras*; establishing credentialing requirements for the individual *promotoras*, their instructors, and the institutions that train them; and suggesting how *promotoras* can be reimbursed within the structure of health care financing.

Lots of changes have taken place since the day I first met Lorenza. The pallet and cardboard houses are gone from the *colonias* near our clinic, and water and sewage lines have been constructed for some of the community. Changes in Medicaid and other programs have made health care more accessible for many residents in the *colonias*. And Lorenza has become successful beyond any expectation I might have had that summer day five years ago. Just recently she was recognized by the Health Care Financing Administration in a public ceremony in New York City. She was lauded for her accomplishments in mobilizing a grassroots effort using *promotoras* to encourage SCHIP enrollment in communities along the entire U.S.–Mexico border.

Yet some things remain the same. My little clinic still operates out of a double-wide mobile home and is the only source of health care for many of the people who come to see me. Family health care for some of my patients is still fragmented between the United States and Mexico. Clinic staff from Texas Tech and the University of Texas at El Paso still depend upon the *promotora* to provide care that we cannot. The current *promotora* in our clinic, like Lorenza, began as a student in one of our clinic classes.

In many respects, the access to health care that most of the rest of the nation enjoys has bypassed the poor people of the border region. But in their own quiet, forceful way, Lorenza and women like her in *colonias* from Texas to California are making the case for community-based health care. The rest of us need to keep working to assure their recognition and support.

⌇ *Immigration Pediatrics*

An inner-city pediatrician finds himself in a medical no-man's land where social policies undermine the care of his newly arrived immigrant patients—and their contributions to society.

Fitzhugh Mullan

I was perplexed. The young woman accompanying the four-year-old to my office for an anemia re-check seemed vague about the child's health and couldn't tell me if he had finished the prescribed course of medication. I suddenly understood. "You're not his mother." "No, I'm not," she told me. "His mother is at work. I'm his sister." She was seventeen years old and

Volume 24, Number 6: 1619–1623. November/December 2005.

understandably uncertain about the child's health, having arrived from El Salvador only ten days before. She spoke no English, was undocumented, and had not enrolled in school. She was just getting to know her mother, whom she hadn't seen in five years, and her young brother, whom she hadn't met before. I examined the child, reordered a blood test, and gave the sister an appointment for an exam—for herself, something she would need before she could go to school.

I practice pediatrics at a community health center in inner-city Washington, D.C., and the reality of immigration is with me every day. A full 90 percent of the children I see are immigrants or the children of immigrants. The majority of them come from Central America or the Caribbean, but Vietnamese, Chinese, and East and West Africans are frequent visitors as well. Although my business card says "pediatrics," in reality I practice immigration medicine.

In college I took a course in U.S. social history. "We are an immigrant nation," our professor told us frequently. "The history of the immigrant is the history of America." I was not convinced. The time was 1963, and immigration history seemed interesting but dated. I had an Irish immigrant grandfather, but to me immigration was mostly stories from the past—stories of families left behind, the ocean voyage in steerage, Ellis Island, Chinese workers building the Transcontinental Railway, and slave ships making the deadly passage from Africa. This was American history, all right, but it was not America as I saw it in the 1960s. I was short-sighted.

New Arrivals and New Citizens

Currently an estimated 1.5 million legal and illegal immigrants arrive in the United States each year. Some 43 percent of immigrant children live in low-income families, and almost one-third do not have health insurance. Each year 750,000 children are born to immigrant women. One way or another, insured or uninsured, sick or well, many of these children pass under the examining hands of pediatricians in a variety of settings, including community health centers such as the one in which I work. Like teachers and social workers, pediatricians constitute an important reception committee for immigrant children in the United States. We are not Hull House or the Henry Street Settlement—well known to earlier immigrants—but we are the conduit to U.S. social services and the first step on the road to becoming Americans. However, like teachers and social workers, we often staff a system that wasn't designed with the best interests of our patients in mind.

Most of the kids I see are the children of Latino immigrants; they were born in the United States and are U.S. citizens. The neighborhood may be dangerous and the schools lousy, but these children are advantaged compared to their immigrant parents and to children arriving here as immigrants. Kids born here grow up speaking English, are entitled to Medicaid, and enter Head Start and the school system with a leg up. I often see families where the five-year-old responds in English and translates for his non-English-speaking parents.

Many Latino immigrant children have a tougher road. War and poverty have driven their parents from Central America to undertake the perilous illegal journey to the United States. These people are often among the most industrious and ambitious in the communities from which they come, men and women intent on finding jobs, saving money, and building families. They staff our restaurants, clean our houses and offices, and labor on our construction sites. Adults usually attempt the trip to the United States alone in the hopes of establishing a safe haven to which they can later bring their children. And they do.

The problem is that to save their families, they pull them apart—at least for a time. The children left behind may get the benefit of money, gifts, and clothes sent home, but they are temporary orphans. Many of the parents in the United States remain "illegal," and when they decide to reunite their families, they have to pay $7,000–$10,000 to cover the costs for human smugglers ("coyotes"), bribes, car, bus, and airfare to get a child to Washington, D.C. Parents with no wherewithal to manage intervening events initiate the trip in the hopes that their child will arrive safely in the United States. It is hard to know what percentage succeed in making the trip since we only see the winners, but many surely fail along the way. Win or lose, these trips are dangerous and expensive.

When these children arrive, they are not eligible for Medicaid or most public assistance. They come to offices like mine for the medical examination and immunizations required to enter school. It is hard to fathom the reunions I regularly see—children raised by a grandmother for ten years suddenly back in the care of their mother. Ten-year-olds entrusted to a stranger to convey them 2,000 miles across three countries for an illegal and uncertain rendezvous with their parents. Teenagers crossing the Sonoran Desert on foot in the hope of finding a ride on an Arizona road that will take them to a bus terminal. There is always a celebratory element to the office visit: "He made it! Wonderful. Congratulations!" But powerfully complex emotions are also going on in the hearts and heads of the children in these reunited families. "Why was I left? How am I going to fit in? Who are these people anyway?"

Newly arrived immigrant children, whether legal or illegal, face the daunting gauntlet of a new school in a new language. Most local schools offer English for speakers of other languages (ESOL) for the newly arrived. While this may work for younger students, youths arriving in high school rarely master English with much proficiency, undoubtedly finding it easier to hang with kids who speak Spanish. Parents are working. City life is fast and rough. The cultural gap can be huge, especially for children from rural communities. I recently cared for a newly arrived seventeen-year-old girl from the countryside of Honduras who had no idea what a condom was or how it was used. The D.C. high school in which she was enrolling has a large infant care center—for the children of students.

More Than a Medical Mission

I do the standard things: looking for undiagnosed problems, testing for parasites, applying TB tests, giving catch-up immunizations, and seeking any signs of abuse or neglect. But my medical mission today is different from what it would have been in earlier times, when malnutrition was the leading problem for immigrant children and blindness-causing trachoma and "imbecility" were considered hazards to the nation. Today the risks for arriving youth are less what they bring with them than what happens after they get here.

Several years ago I examined a fifteen-year-old boy newly arrived from El Salvador who came to the clinic accompanied by his mother. He was nicely dressed, clean-cut—and sullen. The mother looked at me and at the ceiling, but never at him. Six weeks in the U.S, and their ten-year-long dream had come unraveled. Talking with me separately, he told me he couldn't believe she had left him at age five, and she told me he was insolent and didn't appreciate what it had taken to get him here. He had started leaving home in the evening and not returning until the next day. The hostility and disappointment in the room was palpable. Was I watching the end of family life and the start of gang life for this young man? Gangs are large and growing in Washington as in other U.S. cities, providing "community" of a sort for many troubled adolescents and recently arrived youths. Kids like my patient can get recruited quickly and lethally. I talked with him alone about gangs, school, drugs, and violence. He admitted to hanging with gang kids and said that he understood the dangers. He told his mom in my presence that he would try to go to school and come home at night.

I have many patients whose lives have gone badly at junctures like this — fifteen-year-olds brought in for truancy, pregnant fourteen-year-olds, a twelve-year-old hit in the abdomen by a stray bullet from a gang shootout. Medical care puts a floor under these kids' feet, but life on the street and opportunities in school will be key to their futures. The importance of a pediatrician in the life of this young man was my ability to refer him — much as I might have done if he had a heart murmur. The "prescription" I used was the Latin American Youth Center (LAYC), a nearby street-smart, multipurpose, safe haven for teens. The nonprofit LAYC beats gangs at their own game by providing a place to belong, social life, and an identity, as well as educational opportunities and jobs. It is the LAYC and organizations like it that stand the best chance of protecting my patients from gangs, early pregnancy, drugs, AIDS, and jail.

Medical No-Man's Land

Such organizations are few and far between, and gangs are ubiquitous and growing. The robust U.S. economy and the ambitions of poor people from around the world are going to keep the arteries of immigration — legal and illegal — flowing briskly for the foreseeable future. Illegal migration in particular creates special hardships for children, of which broken lives, criminality, and disease are too often the outcome. But as a country, we are schizophrenic about immigrants, welcoming and xenophobic at the same time. We want their energy and their hustle but not their illnesses or their family problems. We consume their labor in huge quantities, but we're not ready to give them jobs with benefits — or have the government make up the difference. Federal welfare and immigration legislation of the mid-1990s imposed a five-year ban on Medicaid eligibility for all nonrefugee immigrants; as a result, new programs such as the State Children's Health Insurance Program (SCHIP) don't reach many of my patients. Jobs without insurance and restrictions in public programs mean that 74 percent less is spent on health care for immigrant children than for kids born in the United States. We want the cheap, flexible, eager muscle of immigrants but not their premature infants, gunshot wounds, or troubled teenagers. As a pediatrician, I often feel as if I labor in a no-man's land between the full-throttle economy and penny-ante social policies.

Fairness, at the least, calls out for change. Reforming immigration laws to give more workers legal status, something the Bush administration has raised as an issue, is the place to begin. This would mean that workers could come and go from the United States without the fear of arrest and deportation, reducing the pressures that drive families apart and decreasing the number of children raised without parents. This is essential to making immigrant life less intrinsically unfriendly to families. But increased medical and social investments in the immigrant community are also essential, both for fairness and to build better citizens for the future. It is well-funded Medicaid and community health center programs, as well as more youth centers and high-quality schools—all at risk in our current public budgets—that will give these new Americans a better chance at success and make our cities safer as well.

The U.S. Supreme Court ruled in 1982 that school systems could not deny undocumented children admission, acknowledging that countenancing children growing up illiterate in America was neither ethical nor in the country's best interests. The same principle needs to be adopted—with the same rationale—for the health care of children. Providing good access for kids to immunizations, controlling infectious diseases, preventing obesity, providing mental health care, and the like will benefit both the immigrant family and the U.S. workforce of the future. Fully funding Medicaid, ending immigrant-specific restrictions on SCHIP eligibility, providing interpreter services where needed, and requiring employer-sponsored insurance coverage for immigrant workers would be the next steps in building a floor under the health of immigrants.

Recently, the sullen fifteen-year-old boy—now nineteen and smiling—came to visit the clinic to show me, amazingly enough, his high school diploma. He had managed to stay off the streets and master his studies well enough to earn a passing grade, a year or so behind schedule. In English that was accented but clear, he explained his plans to work in construction during the day and take some college classes at night. His mother came with him. She was delightfully proud. She told me that she never thought this would happen. Never. I certainly would not have predicted a positive outcome from the unpromising start in the examination room interview several years before. I was pleased for them and happy to have been a small participant in this tiny piece of American history—the boy becoming a man, the Salvadoran becoming an American, medicine as social service, immigration pediatrics.

CHAPTER 8

VALUES AND CHOICE

STORIES OF PRACTICAL ETHICS

⌐ Casey's Legacy

A physician finds generosity when admitting to an error in judgment.

W. RICHARD BOYTE

They were older than I had pictured the parents of a six-month-old infant to be. Appearing small and vulnerable, they sat nervously on the edge of the hard-cushioned vinyl couch. I had spoken with them for the first time by phone four hours earlier. Since then they had traveled by car from their small hometown to the Children's Hospital at the University of Mississippi Medical Center in Jackson. Upon arrival, they had been asked to wait for us in the family conference room. The small space became cramped as the group of doctors, medical students, and nurses entered. After initial greetings, the room became even more uncomfortable as silence filled the remaining space.

As agreed upon, the fellow of cardiovascular surgery cleared his throat to deliver the news to Casey's parents. In a soft voice he said, "I'm so sorry to have to tell you, but Casey died about an hour ago." With his voice dropping to barely above a whisper, he continued, "We tried to get in touch with you but you were already on your way. Remember me telling you how sick she could get with her infection? She was just too, too sick to live. I hope you will understand." I waited for him to go on, but the silence told me he was finished.

Confused and grieving, I felt my distress turn to anguish. Not from what he told them. Not even from the manner in which he did it. Casey may indeed have been too sick to survive. But it was what was not disclosed that added to my distress. A complication occurred in the last minutes of Casey's life during an attempted procedure. This complication was the unintended consequence of medical judgment. However, an error in that judgment created the circumstances that pushed Casey's life beyond saving. A physician made that error. I was that physician.

Volume 20, Number 2: 250–254. March/April 2001.

Casey was born with congenital heart disease to parents in their late forties who live in one of the poorest areas of rural Mississippi. They were of limited financial means, but their love for their daughter appeared unlimited. At six months of age, however, Casey appeared frail and undernourished. Despite the best efforts of the medical staff, Casey's parents never appeared to have more than a basic understanding of her heart defect. They also lacked a reliable means of transportation, which resulted in Casey's missing several of her appointments. As a result, a surgical repair that could have been performed earlier in infancy had been delayed until fourteen days before her death.

The surgical repair itself went very well. Casey's parents had been told that their infant's poor state of health would place her at high risk for complications. Nonetheless, they were given an optimistic report shortly after the surgery. They soon returned to their home and were kept updated by phone of their daughter's progress. Casey continued to require mechanical ventilation because her heart had developed very poor function. Then pneumonia set in, progressing rapidly to sepsis syndrome with widespread toxic effects. Her condition became extremely fragile. As a pediatric critical care specialist, I was consulted to help.

Casey's kidneys soon failed. A pediatric nephrologist recommended a supportive therapy called hemofiltration to partially replace the function of the kidneys. Through this measure, retained fluid might be removed from the infant's body. But as I examined the pale, limp, swollen figure before me, I questioned the effectiveness of the proposed therapy. Her prognosis was extremely poor with or without this procedure. Only a slim chance existed that she would survive at all. The associated complications of the therapy would be especially dangerous in this critically ill infant.

Good Intentions

Despite the bleak outlook for Casey's life, my desire to help her began to quickly overcome my misgivings. I became convinced that the recommended supportive therapy could prove instrumental in her survival. We required a central venous catheter; one was already in use in a femoral vein, but we would need a separate one. Casey's attending physician, a cardiovascular surgeon, was informed. He also agreed that hemofiltration might give Casey a chance to survive. Casey's parents, of course, would have to give their permission.

I contacted Casey's parents by phone, carefully explaining the proposed supportive therapy. Then I described the procedure that would put into place the central venous catheter: A needle is used to locate a large vein; through the needle a long wire can be introduced into the blood vessel. The catheter, a long tube, is then placed into the vein over the wire. I explained that, in Casey's critical condition, this procedure could be risky. I described the possible complications carefully. They asked few questions and made few comments. Before giving her permission, Casey's mother told me that she always trusted the doctors to do what was best for Casey.

I chose the subclavian vein that lies under the right collarbone for the catheter site. I did so because a chest tube was already positioned in Casey's right chest cavity. This tube had been in place since shortly after surgery, to drain fluid from around the lung. My hope was that the chest tube would also drain any blood or air unintentionally produced during my attempt to locate the subclavian vein. This air or blood could otherwise collect around the lung and cause its collapse.

My first pass with the needle produced no result. Typically, an aspiration of dark blood into the syringe attached to the needle indicates that the vein has been located. But on my second pass, when a brief flash of bright red blood came into the syringe, I realized that I had inadvertently punctured the subclavian artery. Seconds later, I noticed the same colored blood coming through the chest tube. I knew there was a chance for bleeding to become persistent and difficult to control. I nervously watched the chest tube. The flow of bright red blood was short-lived. I felt some relief but continued to watch Casey's monitor for changes in her vital signs. I listened closely to compare the intensity of breath sounds over both sides of the chest. Eventually convincing myself that the bleeding had stopped, I returned to the task of finding the subclavian vein.

Losing Casey

I was leaning over the baby when the monitor alarm was triggered by her rapidly rising heart rate. Pulling back the small sterile drape used for the procedure, I saw that Casey now appeared ashen white. Her blood pressure began to rapidly fall. With rising alarm, I looked down to her side at the chest tube. No new blood could be seen draining through it. As I reached for a stethoscope, Casey's heart rate began to plummet. The nurse started chest compressions. Through the stethoscope, I discovered too late that lung sounds were now diminished over the right side of Casey's chest. A new chest tube released a large amount of fresh blood.

Despite a prolonged effort to save Casey, her fragile heart, once stopped, would not beat again. A clot in the original chest tube had hidden the bleeding that filled Casey's chest. Casey's weak grip on life was loosened. I can still vividly remember the wave of nausea and pounding in my temples as I looked at her gray, lifeless face.

In the five years since this incident, I have thought of Casey often. Recently I had cause to think of her again as I read a critique of the Institute of Medicine's (IOM's) 1999 report, *To Err Is Human*. The report stated that medical errors cause between 44,000 and 98,000 deaths annually in U.S. hospitals. Not surprisingly, the report has faced a mostly cool reception from the medical community, which has questioned its accuracy. Nonetheless, calls for measures to prevent adverse events are now abundant. If nothing else, the medical community is being compelled to take the same difficult inward look that I took five years ago.

Doctors find it difficult to admit mistakes, especially mistakes in judgment. In this case, my desire to help Casey caused me to overreach. I wonder now how many of the errors estimated in the IOM report are made under similar circumstances. In my own case, I hope that acknowledging a tendency to overreach has prevented me from repeating such errors. This is Casey's legacy to me.

Telling the Truth

Casey's father sat in silence, softly caressing his wife's hand. She cried quietly. The dignity and grace with which they accepted the news of their daughter's death moved me. As I looked into the faces of Casey's parents, I thought of many reasons to maintain my silence. I wondered if the cardiovascular fellow was reciting the same reasons to himself. He likely felt that by not telling them what happened, he was performing a kindness both to me and to Casey's parents. This way, I would not have to admit that a complication occurred. In addition, their confidence in the medical care that their daughter received would not be disturbed. I told myself that Casey, after all, would likely have died with or without the planned therapy. Furthermore, the complication was not unanticipated. A hemothorax is a known complication to the procedure we attempted. In fact, I had warned them that such a life-threatening complication could occur. I took appropriate precautions, and I addressed the threat to her life immediately. I told myself that fuller disclosure would not bring Casey back to life.

I reasoned that I had not been negligent to them or to Casey. I also reasoned that I had only the best of intentions for their daughter. However, as I watched them rise from their seats, I also began to admit to myself that an error had occurred. I had made a human error pursuing the noblest of human intentions: to save a life. Despite this intent, I had erred in my medical judgment that this was a highly necessary option in Casey's management. Perhaps a different outcome would have occurred if I had judged the procedure for the central venous catheter (as well as hemofiltration itself) to be too risky for Casey. I will never know with any high degree of certainty.

As they started to go I stopped them. "Wait," I said, "There's more."

I paused to collect my thoughts and then said, "It's true that Casey was probably too sick to live. But I should tell you more about how her life ended." With that, I proceeded to describe the last moments of their daughter's life. It took just a few minutes. I explained as well as I could what happened. I told them about the hemothorax and the clot in the chest tube. I can still recall the mixture of relief and embarrassment. After another pause, I slowly and carefully explained to them how it might have been a mistake to choose a more aggressive approach to Casey's medical management. When I finally fell silent they stared blankly through me. After a long moment they asked if they could see their daughter.

I walked some distance behind them as they entered the pediatric intensive care unit. I watched as they stepped behind the faded, dingy curtain that was pulled around Casey's bed. I sat quietly within the safety of the nurse's station. I wanted to leave. No, I wanted to run. Even so, I felt an obligation to stay in case they had questions. Why did I tell them so much? Was I seeking some form of absolution? Perhaps so, but I hope my true purpose in full disclosure was, in the end, more honorable. They had entrusted me with their daughter's life. I owed them the truth.

Eventually, they reemerged from behind the curtain. When it seemed they would walk past me in silence, I was both disappointed and relieved. But they suddenly stopped. Casey's father held out his hand. I held out mine, which trembled as he gripped it. In a quiet, firm voice he said, "Thank you, doctor, for trying to help my daughter." Afterward, Casey's mother accepted my embrace.

⌒ No One Needs to Know

A physician recalls taking part in his first cover-up.

Neil S. Calman

M
y indoctrination into the underworld of medical secrecy began twenty-five years ago during my first clinical rotation in my third year of medical school. The lessons learned were not a formal part of my medical school curriculum but are as indelibly etched into my brain as are the names of the body parts I studied in anatomy.

The voyage began with the care of a patient I will call Charles McNight. Just over sixty years old, he had come to the medical center to receive the care of our most highly skilled cardiovascular surgeons. They replaced two of his heart valves, put a graft on his aorta, and performed bypass surgery—all in one procedure. I do not recall the details of his cardiac pathology, but he sailed through the surgery, and his rapid recovery far exceeded our expectations.

I had gotten to know "Charlie" because I had been assigned to do his admitting history and physical, a typical job in those days for medical students. His thick, pure white, Santa-like beard and the warm smile beneath it instantly charmed all who met him. His wife and daughter were equally engaging. I became rapidly and intensely involved in his care, providing a human touch—a role that medical students often play on the hospital team in lieu of making medical decisions for which they are not yet prepared.

Crossing Boundaries

My care for Charlie was both fueled and complicated by my infatuation with his daughter, who was my age and unmarried. Her life as a single parent of a four-year-old daughter gave me ample substrate on which to build a wonderful fantasy. It was simple, it seemed, to help bring Charlie home, get him

Volume 20, Number 2: 243–249. March/April 2001.

well, fall in love with his daughter, and be a stepfather to her little girl. These fantasies kept me returning to his hospital room.

A few weeks after surgery, Charlie was ready to be discharged. He went home with instructions to return weekly to the hospital lab for blood tests needed to adjust his level of coumarin, a medicine he was taking to prevent blood clots. A few days after discharge I received a call from his wife inviting me to their home for dinner—a small way for them to thank me for the extra care I had given Charlie in the hospital. I accepted, yet acknowledged to myself my level of discomfort in doing so. I had clearly crossed the line I had been taught to maintain between doctor and patient; I had allowed myself to become personally involved in Charlie's life. Dinner took place almost a week after Charlie's discharge, and I offered to bring the necessary equipment to take his required blood tests and to transport the blood back to the hospital lab. Charlie was grateful; he lived quite a distance from the hospital and was not looking forward to making the trip.

Dinner was great. Afterward, Charlie and I went into another room where I drew his blood. I then excused myself for the evening. The results of the tests were fine, and Charlie was doing well until a few weeks later, when he began to experience some sweats and weakness and the sensation that something was going wrong. Hours later he developed a low-grade fever that, within twelve hours, raged to 104 degrees. He called me at home that night. I was very worried for him and told him to go immediately to the hospital. His wife helped him put on a robe, and Charlie left home for what would be the last time.

I lived only a few blocks from the hospital and arrived almost an hour before Charlie and his wife. I was exhausted by my anxiety. My rotation in cardiovascular surgery had since ended, so I was there as a friend—a role I was not supposed to be playing as a medical student. Yet I was clearly part of the institution that was now responsible for Charlie's life.

Charlie's wife pulled their car into the emergency entrance. I helped him in to the hospital. Sweat was beading on his brow; he was so weak he could hardly stand. I took one of his hands in mine. It was cold and wet from perspiration. My other hand gently touched his back to support him; even through his robe and two shirts I could feel the thermal struggle his body was waging against some unknown infectious invader. Within moments it became clear to the cardiac surgery fellow on call that Charlie had an infection, and all too clear about its probable cause. "I am admitting you to the hospital in intensive care," he told Charlie, whose face looked close to death. "You have an infection, maybe on your aortic graft."

Slippery Slope

A shudder went through me. I had seen two similar cases while on the cardiovascular surgery service. In both cases patients had been discharged from the hospital, had returned with fever, and died. I had also heard that there might have been a problem with a batch of cardiovascular catheters that were in use in the hospital. Weeks after use, some had been suspected to have been contaminated, presumably by the manufacturer, with a fungus called candida. The patients who had been catheterized with these units were subject to postoperative infection with the fungus and seemed to be resistant to treatment.

By morning the surgical team that originally treated Charlie was by his bedside. Only one hope remained: They loaded him with antifungal drugs and took him to surgery to replace the infected graft. I changed my clothes and went into the operating room to watch. The thought of being able to answer his family's questions about the long and complex surgery was so powerful that it obscured the pain that developed in my feet as I stood, out of the way, on a tiny patch of floor in the OR.

The surgery went well and confirmed the infection. Charlie was back in the cardiosurgical intensive care unit, and I was by his bedside with his wife and daughter. The surgeon appeared shortly thereafter and briefly reassured the family that his team had replaced the infected graft and that Charlie had done very well in surgery. The surgeon walked away. I stood with Charlie's wife and daughter and explained what I could about what I had seen in the OR, leaving out any mention that the infection he had suffered might have been caused by the contaminated catheters. Minutes later, a bell sounded, indicating the end of visiting hours. I left with them as if the bell was meant for me, too, and sat in the waiting area discussing with them my optimism about Charlie's future.

As Pavlovian as the family's response to the visiting hours bell, my response to the hospital's emergency paging system was equally well programmed. I had learned since starting my clinical rotations that the moment a voice began to ring out on the pager, all other incoming auditory signals were instinctively shut out. The "code" was called for the cardiac surgical intensive care unit. I froze in fear, listening to the announcement. I told Charlie's family I needed to respond to this, a total fabrication, and left. The crowd around Charlie's bed confirmed my fears.

I was immobilized by not knowing what to do, by my emotions, and by the people running in every direction with medications and equipment. A few minutes later the surgeon who had just completed Charlie's graft repair came to the bedside. There was no hope. All resuscitation attempts failed to restart his heart. As the code was called to a halt, a nurse hurriedly handed a STAT lab result to the surgeon. The patient's serum potassium had soared to a level that would have made anyone's heart stop. I looked over the surgeon's shoulder as he held the slip of paper with the lab result, staring in disbelief. Charlie had died of a simple mistake. His potassium had been allowed to go too high after surgery. This well-known deadly event was caused by the release of large amounts of potassium into the blood from cells damaged at surgery. The event is so common in cardiac surgical procedures that close monitoring of the potassium was a routine part of postoperative care. How could such a small oversight undo the months of heroic medical care that Charlie had been given by the most skilled surgeons in the region?

Entering the Dungeon of Deception

The surgeon looked at me and to my great surprise put his arm around my shoulder. I was unaware that he had given a moment's thought to my role in Charlie's care. "Son," he began, "I've been very moved by the interest and concern you have shown for this patient. I also know that you realize that nothing good would come out of the family's knowing about the catheter problems or what happened just now. No one needs to know." He tapped my shoulder twice and walked away.

In those few seconds it happened. I had been invited to join the underworld of medical secrecy—that territory where doctors tread and where no others may look in; where secrets about mistakes and problems are brought and where they reside forever hidden.

I stood motionless. A stream of contradictory thoughts flooded my brain. Was I Charlie's friend, and should friendship prevail? Should I tell his family everything I knew? Or was I a doctor, albeit in training, committed to keeping the secrets that lie beyond the patients' and families' grasp? Was I partially responsible for the future survival of the wife, daughter, and granddaughter Charlie had left behind? Had I done everything I could? I had lit- tle time to think, and I never really made a decision what to do. The surgeon left my side and went to the waiting room to tell the news to Charlie's wife and daughter. I knew I had to follow but didn't know if I should be standing next to the family or next to the doctor.

The surgeon offered his condolences to the family. He remained only briefly and then asked if I could stay with them for a while. He was depu- tizing me — an act that subconsciously sucked me deeper into the under- world. I was now responsible for maintaining the charade that "we had done everything we could." It was up to me to understand the importance of the statement, "No one needs to know."

I saw Charlie's family only once after that, at his funeral. His daughter in- troduced me to everyone there as one of Charlie's doctors who had taken such good care of him. I played the role well. Dressed in my only suit, I told them how much he had endured, how sick he had been, and how he kept all of our spirits high to the end.

I got in my car and drove home across the city in a pouring rain. That was the last time I saw Charlie's family. I could not remain in contact with them while being filled with the secrets I had been implored not to reveal: the con- taminated catheters that might have caused his infection, and the elevated potassium level that caused his heart to stop beating. I would be living a lie each moment I spent with his family. Even the closeness I had felt to them, my thoughts of his daughter, and my continuing sense of responsibility for them were not strong enough to overcome my discomfort. I knew I could not violate the laws of the secret society of medicine into which I had just begun my initiation. Being invited into the sanctity of this dungeon of de- ception was part of the honor of becoming a doctor. It made me feel spe- cial — an entrusted colleague, a real doctor. But many questions flooded my mind.

Had anyone else died before Charlie as the result of fatally high potas- sium after surgery? Had anyone explored the need to change the systems by which such monitoring took place? Did the company that made the catheters know that some had been contaminated? Would lawsuits have forced them out of business, making these devices unavailable to others who would benefit? Would the hospital be forced to pay millions to those who died as a result, eroding the services it was providing to other patients? Would doctors be afraid to assume the challenges of critically ill patients like Charlie? Did Charlie's family deserve to be compensated for the errors that caused their loss? Would the benefits to that one family outweigh the damage that could be done to the physicians and the hospital?

I had no answers and thus did nothing. Today I am puzzled by how quickly I adapted to this new role of "keeper of secrets" and remain concerned that others entering medicine are still taught in the same way.

Unstated Obstacles to Openness

What keeps any doctor I have ever known from initiating discussion of medical mistakes with patients is a set of redoubtable barriers. First, there is tacit agreement among physicians that mistakes are an inevitable part of practicing medicine. I have made my own errors over the years, some with minor adverse outcomes, others with horrible results. When I discover another physician's mistake, I only discuss it if the doctor is employed by me or is formally under my supervision. We physicians are afraid to turn up the heat on others lest we fry in our own fire.

Then we have the specter of medical liability lawsuits. Who would reveal errors to a patient and initiate the years-long process of defending a medical liability lawsuit? The financial burden of such an action and the public humiliation involved are insurmountable for most physicians and deter a more honest reckoning of medical errors among physicians and between physicians and patients.

Finally, like most doctors, I went into medicine to be a helper and healer. Scrutiny by colleagues and the process of discussing my mistakes openly with others compel me to relive, over and over, the pain of having played a role in injuring someone who entrusted me with his or her life. A prolonged probing of my errors would force a level of self-doubt that would affect future decisions and could prove immobilizing. With no grounds for comparing my abilities and practice skills with those of my colleagues, I would be left asking, "Do I make more mistakes than my colleagues? Would another doctor have done a better job taking care of this patient?"

The formal internal quality assurance discussions that have been implemented in some institutions take place in a protected environment and thus promote a more open review of the cause of medical errors. Such sheltered examination often results in fixing systemic problems and thereby protecting patients from a simple oversight like the one that killed Charlie Mc-

Night. But building a legal firewall between quality review processes and public scrutiny fails to create a mechanism for the legitimate compensation of patients who have been injured through medical mistakes. Studies have shown that only a small percentage of such injuries are compensated through legal actions, while most go unaddressed.

The process by which law and medicine have evolved to deal with medical mistakes must be drastically changed, both to compensate those injured and to encourage the disclosure of errors. At the same time, each of us, as physicians and teachers, must fight the continuing urge to hide our mistakes. We must teach the next generation of students to talk about medical errors as a part of medical practice that will always be with us. Most of all, we must teach each other that the biggest gaffe of all is to cover up our mistakes, thus perpetuating barriers to safe care.

Everyone needs to know.

∽ At the End of a Day

A young doctor considers an end-of-life decision and the love that informs it.

ALOK KHORANA

It's four o'clock in the afternoon and I'm sort of tired. Not physically tired, just tired of being at work at the hospital. I've been saving up vacation time, and it must finally be getting to me. I sit down at the nurses' station to take a break. I've been on the go for the past nine hours, but I'm close to being caught up. I rummage through my overflowing lab coat pocket and drag out my "census." When I'm on the floors, this worn, crumpled sheet is my life-blood—my list of patients. Each morning it starts out as a neat, computer-generated list. By the end of the day, as now, multiple, barely decipherable scribbles appear around each name. I scan quickly through the

Volume 22, Number 6: 239–243. November/December 2003. This narrative is a short story and its characters are fictional.

list, pleased at the crossed-out Ls and Os next to each patient. In my short-hand, this means that labs have been checked and orders written. The un-crossed N next to twelve names means I only need to write twelve notes, then I'll be caught up.

This isn't so bad, I think, glancing at my watch. At five minutes a note, I should be done by five o'clock, and that'll still give me an hour to spare be-fore my call's done. Fully motivated now, I square my shoulders, pick up a pen, and arrange the charts in front of me. The nurse standing at the end of the counter reminds me of what I've been trying not to think about. "Have you been practicing your 'I do's'?" she asks, smirking. I smile back politely, not wanting to respond. "One day more before it's all over, you know," she continues, ignoring my lack of interest in this conversation. "Just one more day." It's not really a day, it's a day and a half: tonight, after work, and all day tomorrow. That's how much time left before I get married.

Hoping to avoid more wisecracks, I start to write my first note of the day. Usually I'm doing this at eleven in the morning, which tells you what kind of day I've had. I try to recapture my motivation, although my train of thought is now running on tracks I've been successful at evading all day. It's five past four, and I'm still hoping to get out on time.

That hope lasts all of ten minutes. As I extend my hand for chart number three on my list, I see Ann moving purposefully toward me. She smiles as she deposits faxed copies of a medical chart on the counter in front of me. "Please, Ann . . . don't tell me," I say. Ann's the charge nurse, so this must be a "direct"—a patient being admitted from a doctor's office, without an emergency room workup, which means extra work for the person on the floor doing the admis-sion—me. "It's worse than you think," she says, as I leaf through the paperwork.

The initial consult note from six months ago tells me most of the story: white male, fifty-three, Vietnam vet, steel plant worker, smoker, lung can-cer—widely metastatic at diagnosis. As I rummage through more clinic notes, I find that he's failed two different chemotherapy regimens and his last few scans have shown an impressive disease progression. At the bottom of the pile I find a handwritten note faxed today from his doctor's office: cough, severe shortness of breath, low oxygen saturations; needs urgent admission. In other words, he's dying and it'll be easier on everybody if he dies in a hospital. I look back up at her. "He should be on hospice." She shrugs in reply; she has seen this before, and, after a while, some battles are not worth fighting. "He's in complete denial; won't even consider a DNR," she says. I groan. This is every physician's nightmare. A dying patient who hasn't had time to adjust, refuses to acknowledge the obvious, so won't sign the Do Not Resuscitate form. Worse still, a dying patient who's not mine, with whom I have no relationship, but who will die on my watch within hours of our first meeting.

This, obviously, is not good. "Family?" I ask. "Just a wife," says Ann. "Kids?" She shakes her head. "You don't have any empty rooms," I point out, grasping at straws now. This is futile, but I really don't want this, not tonight. I just want to get out of here. "We transferred someone out to make space for him," Ann replies, smiling mirthlessly.

I give up, resigned to my fate, and return to my paperwork. Within a few minutes there's a commotion by the front desk as a gurney comes down the hallway. It's carrying a half-dressed, middle-aged man, his face half hidden by an oxygen mask. He's escorted by two paramedics and accompanied by the stench of desperation. Instinctively, I glance at the clock on the wall—twenty past four. He's already here; with that goes my last chance of getting out of this mess. (There's no way I can convince the night on-call doctor that the patient came in at "almost" five o'clock.)

I walk up as the nurses shift him onto his bed. His head is bald, the mark of Cain for a chemotherapy patient. His face is flushed, nostrils flared. He glances toward me as I approach, eyes flicking over the letters "MD" at the end of my name badge, and nods in greeting. "How are you, Mr. Kohl?" I ask, realizing how inane my forced cheeriness must sound. "Not so good, doc," he replies, grimacing as he's lifted onto his bed. Every breath is an effort—the spaces between his ribs filling in and out, pectorals, intercostals, and phrenic nerves working in concert to expand his failing chest, respiratory centers in overdrive, as his body gasps for oxygen. What has come naturally all his life is now gritty, sapping work. And failure is close: The tips of his fingers are blue, so even this monumental effort, mounted by every last cell in his body—normal and malignant—is not succeeding.

He firmly grips my arm. "You're gonna make me all better now, aren't you?" This is a possible opening, but I need to build a relationship here, so I evade the issue. "We'll try, sir," I reply. The room around me has been busy with assorted nurses and aides, hooking up oxygen cannulas, measuring vital signs. I join the fracas and start with a history and physical. Given his condition, my exam is brief and interrupted by various directions to the nurses. "Normal saline is fine, yes, six liters oxygen, nebulizers, call respiratory, yes, of course, he needs telemetry, he's not . . ." Pause. ". . . You know." Not a

DNR, I mean, and they know it, so I don't complete the sentence. Opening number two, but the patient hasn't sensed it, and I let it slide again. The next hour passes swiftly as I finish up the paperwork. Finally, I call the attending physician and explain the situation. "He needs to be DNR," she tells me. I know, I know.

I reenter the patient's room, his chart in my hand, and sit by his bedside. Mr. Kohl opens his eyes and looks tiredly at me. Over his head, the telemetry monitor flickers with new numbers every few seconds, announcing his heart rate, respiratory rate, oxygen saturation. None of those numbers looks good. "We need to talk, Mr. Kohl," I say; that gets his attention. I start by explaining what we've done—the oxygen, the fluids, the monitors. Then I talk about his history, the recent diagnosis, how chemotherapy hadn't worked very well, the increasing number of pulmonary nodules showing on each scan. Finally, I talk about his most recent studies, how much the cancer had advanced, how it was the large tumor nodules that were affecting his breathing, not fluid or pneumonia. There didn't seem to be a lot we could do, except keep him comfortable and pain-free. And, if he wished, we would avoid artificial ventilation, cardiac resuscitation, breathing machines, and electric paddles. Those wouldn't be too comfortable, I told him, and certainly wouldn't do anything for the cancer itself.

He seems to have understood me but doesn't respond, so I bring up the last part again, about not wanting to be resuscitated and signing a DNR form. His hand reaches out and grabs me by the wrist, "No . . . no DNR . . . I'm not giving up, doc, I told my wife, I want everything done!" He falls back, releasing my wrist, his face even more flushed, his neck veins engorged with effort, his face covered with fear. I start over, this time using a different tone, a little harsher, with words like morphine, dying, and even futile. Ann has been standing behind me and pipes in as well. She reminds him of the talks he had with his physician the last time he was in, of the other end-of-life discussions he's had. She speaks firmly of dying with dignity and letting go. Mr. Kohl isn't buying, though. He shakes his head and repeats, "No DNR . . . my wife knows." The fear of death and the will to live are primal human instincts, honed, in this man, over years of working in a steel plant, scarred by serving in 'Nam. He will not be dissuaded by a young trainee doctor with a foreign accent and a nurse who might just be trying to save her hospital some money.

Ann and I retreat to the nurses' station. It is now 8:30. "I'd think a peaceful last call before you leave for your wedding and honeymoon isn't asking too much, but I guess not," she says. I shrug my shoulders and change the subject. "Speaking of marriage, where's his wife?" I ask. "On her way in," Ann replies. "She's a manager at an Applebee's; I called her and explained the situation. She claims she's raised end-of-life issues with him before, but he hasn't wanted to talk about it, and she hasn't pressed the subject." I sit down again and resume working on my notes. There's no rush now. Within the next hour or so he'll crash, and we'll have to intubate him and attach him to a ventilator. He'll stay on it for the next few weeks in an intensive care unit, hooked to central lines and artificial feeds, paralyzed, in considerable physical distress, until his wife and extended family finally decide, with considerable emotional distress, to "pull the plug." This is a lose-lose situation.

It takes me an hour and a half to finish my notes and Mr. Kohl's paperwork, call my attending back, and let the night on-call person in on what's happening. I cross off the last "N" on my list and prepare to leave. As if on cue, the telemetry alarms go off, softly—*ding ding ding*. We all rush into Mr. Kohl's room. He is dropping his oxygen saturations even further, and his respiratory distress is painful to see. I ask the nurse to switch him to the most oxygen we can give him without mechanical ventilation. A code blue has been broadcast overhead, and the room is suddenly full of busy residents, nurses, aides, a respiratory therapist. An officious-looking older nurse stands guard over the code cart outside the room. The anesthesiologist is here now, intubation kit in hand. The bed is pushed down to make room at the head, part of a drill all of us know well. There is comfort, a somber familiarity, in the practiced ease with which such professionals perform. There are times when what we in this room do might actually mean the difference between life and death. Tonight, though, we are merely actors rehearsing for another night and another patient.

I lean over to check one last time with the patient. "Your lungs can't keep up the work, Mr. Kohl, so we'll have to hook you up to a breathing machine. You did say that was what you wanted, right?" This is his last opening, one last chance to say no, to tell us what he really thinks of us, to say that he's had enough, and none of it has worked—not the chemotherapy, the scans, all the attention tonight. It's his last chance to say that he'd like to be left alone with his wife and dog, if he has one, to die in peace, in his own home, in his own bed, with whatever dignity his tired, battered body can muster. "Yes," he rasps from behind the oxygen mask.

"Now, Bob." I turn at the sound of a strange voice. She's standing next to me, a fifty-something woman, looking strangely incongruous in her colorful restaurant uniform, her badge with "Rita: 11 years of serving you" still on her chest. She has short, sandy brown hair, and glasses, and she's slightly over-weight. She has a gold band on her left hand, thin and weather-beaten, a tes-tament to years of service of another kind. I, who have been wondering about marriage, wonder about theirs: How many years? Where are the children? What were your good times, your bad times, your regrets, your joys? In the end, and this is the end, is it worth it? I say none of this, though, as I step back to give her some space. She moves in closer, resting slightly on the edge of the bed, her hand firmly linked to his. Despite the hubbub of activity, the room is strangely silent. I hear her say to him, with pauses for emphasis, "It's . . . OK . . . Bobby." It's all she says, and just once. He looks back at her and then, between gasps of air, tries to shrug his shoulders, as if to say "I tried." Then she turns to me and says, "He doesn't want any of this. Can't you just make him comfortable, doctor?" I look to him for affirmation, and he nods. "Yes, ma'am," I say.

The rest is easy. The anesthesiologist, the respiratory therapist, the ancil-lary personnel all start to leave. A chair is found for Mrs. Kohl, and she sits down next to him, her hand still firmly clasped to his. The monitor is switched off. The morphine orders are written and a drip started. Mr. Kohl's respirations are not quite as agonized as he starts to drift toward sleep. The nurses will try to keep him as comfortable as possible. Once again I inform my attending and the night on-call physician. Finally, I write one last note in the chart. Now I can leave.

By the time I get home it's almost midnight. I curse softly as I stub my toe against an empty moving box lying in the middle of the living room. In the dark I see silhouettes of half-empty moving boxes scattered throughout the apartment and realize that tonight was the night I was supposed to help my fiancée move in. She must have started already, because most of the stuff ap-pears unpacked. She's lying on my bed, asleep. I undress quietly and slide into bed beside her. She stirs quietly but doesn't awaken. As my eyes adjust, I look at her white skin glowing in the dark, the tousled hair, the curve of her shoulder, the long eyelashes fluttering in dream as she sleeps trustfully.

The alarm clock on the nightstand informs me that it is now five minutes into a brand new day. Tomorrow we will be married. Together we'll raise a family, change jobs, move, grow old, and go through life's struggles like a billion other families on the planet—like Rita and Bob. One day I will be dying, and she will come in and tell me it's OK to die. I'll listen to her. And it will be OK.

⌒ *Life but No Limb*

The Aftermath of Medical Error

Money helps, but it's not the sole reason that family members sue.

CAROL LEVINE

This is a story about living with, not dying from, the consequences of medical error. It began in January 1990 when my husband suffered a devastating brain-stem injury in an auto accident on an icy highway in upstate New York. He was driving; we were both wearing seat belts. The car hit a patch of black ice, skidded, hit a guard rail, rolled over, and landed in a deep gully. I emerged shaken but unharmed. My husband was unconscious and unresponsive. In that brief moment our lives changed forever.

I have written about my experiences as my husband's caregiver but have avoided writing, even talking, about the medical error that occurred early in his hospitalization. It is only now, nearly thirteen years later, that I am cautiously ready to tell that part of the story. It is my story because the person to whom direct harm was done is unable to give his own account. The choice to write about such a painful experience brings up feelings of shock, disbelief, and even guilt. In some illogical way, writing about the medical mistake is an embarrassment, as if by doing so I will be exposed to the world as a person whom fate has singled out for a particularly nasty break.

Yet I have overcome these doubts in order to add a different perspective

Volume 21, Number 4: 237–241. July/August 2002. Adapted from a presentation to a meeting of the Medicine as a Profession Forum, a project cosponsored by the United Hospital Fund and the Open Society Institute.

to the oddly disembodied, professional discussion of medical error. Medical error is more than an engineering problem, amenable to technological and "systems" solutions. Policies put in place to reduce medical error also must address the financial and emotional needs of those who suffer great and often permanent harm.

"There Was a Mistake"

After the accident my husband was brought by ambulance to a community hospital. The neurologist on call somberly told me that even if my husband survived, he would be seriously impaired, both cognitively and physically. I wanted another opinion. Despite bad weather and telephone outages, I managed to get my husband transferred to a major New York City tertiary care hospital that same day. There the high priest of neurosurgery vigorously reassured me that my husband would be "one hundred percent okay." So, of course I believed him, not the community hospital doctor, whose initial prognosis turned out to be right.

A week into my husband's stay in the ICU, when he still showed no signs of coming out of the coma, I received a call in the middle of the night from the neurosurgery resident. He said that my husband had a blood clot in his right hand and needed immediate surgery. At the hospital, the plastic surgeon called in on the case assured me that clots like this occur frequently; an operation would clear it out. He said they would give my husband a big dose of heparin to make sure that the clot didn't recur.

The first surgery did not do the job, so back my husband went to the OR in less than twenty-four hours. At that point, the neurosurgeon met me in the hall. He seemed very angry. "There was a mistake," he said. "The catheter used to measure arterial gases became clogged, and a new catheter was placed on the same hand instead of the other hand. You never put two sticks in one hand. When that catheter became clogged, circulation was blocked through his hand."

He then said, "It wasn't noticed for twenty-four hours," the passive voice subtly deflecting responsibility from a human agent. I can quote this line verbatim because it was repeated many times by family members who were there. At the time, though, I saw only the doctor's mouth moving and his hand indicating where the catheter was placed; it was like watching a TV scene with the sound muted. He then said, "They'll fix it. It's not life-threatening." I asked, "But it is hand-threatening, isn't it?" He only shrugged and walked away.

Only later did I remember that on the day before the first surgery, I had told the ICU nurse that my husband's right hand was very cold. She said, "I'll put on another blanket." That brief exchange haunts me to this day. Why didn't I insist that she look at his hand and call a doctor right away? Would it have made a difference? I will never know.

Several surgeries followed, each accompanied by larger and larger doses of heparin. Then came a final, middle-of-the night surgery, after which the plastic surgeon told me, "We can't save his hand. He developed an overwhelming allergic reaction to heparin. Instead of clearing the clot, the heparin made his blood clot so quickly that we couldn't even begin to clear the vessels." I first asked whether this was a systemic reaction. Yes, he replied, but my husband would survive. I then asked whether his hand had been amputated. No, they wanted to wait to see how high up on his arm the damage went.

From Bad to Worse

For the next several days I sat by my husband's bed watching his hand, then his wrist, then his forearm turn black. Suddenly he developed a serious infection and needed emergency surgery, to which I consented. What else could I do? His right forearm was amputated an inch or so below the elbow. For the next several weeks I sat by his side looking at the raw, finally healing stump.

Four months later my husband, still in a coma, was transferred to a rehabilitation facility. Gradually he came out of the coma, disoriented, confused, and incontinent. He was unable to sit up, eat, or move without assistance. The brain stem controls these functions; his was irreparably damaged. When he began to recognize me and understand a little of what happened, he repeatedly asked me to put his wheelchair in front of a mirror. He believed that his lost arm had been placed somewhere else on his body and that I was not showing him where it was.

The psychologist on staff was sympathetic, but from the beginning the rehabilitation therapists dismissed any possibility that my husband could use his right arm in any functional way. In the acute care hospital the specialists had assured me that with new prosthetic materials and therapy, my husband would be able to do almost everything he did before—go back to his job as a public relations executive, give presentations, everything. Upset by the re-habilitation therapists' appraisal, I called the original doctors and asked for a consultation. No one responded. My husband never got a prosthesis that provided any functional benefit, and he scorned the one that was supposed to look like a normal hand.

At this point—and only at this point—I started to get mad. Not only had my husband's prognosis for meaningful recovery been wildly overstated, but he had suffered a terrible loss and no one seemed to care. What would he have been able to do with a right arm intact? Hard to know. He was, in ef-fect, paralyzed, but he was extremely sensitive to touch, which made physi-cal therapy painful. His left hand was useless. Perhaps with a stronger right hand he could have fed himself, turned the pages of a book, changed the channels on the TV, helped in transfers from bed to wheelchair, touched me, and held our grandchildren. These are not meaningless actions in his life or mine.

Looking to the Law

A prominent corporate attorney I knew was trying to get our insurance com-pany to cover some home care. He offered to talk to the hospital adminis-tration off the record and try to get a small settlement for us. No one at the hospital would return his calls, and then he too started to get mad.

As the deadline for filing a lawsuit approached, he urged me to think about this option. Our future was bleak. My husband's health insurer had paid for all of the care associated with the medical error—amounting to sev-eral hundred thousand dollars—and we were rapidly reaching the cap on his policy. Moreover, insurance coverage for home care would be very lim-ited. To keep my husband at home and my life reasonably intact, I would have to pay for his care myself.

I had no idea how to find a responsible malpractice attorney, because all I had ever heard from my health care colleagues was the usual badmouthing of trial lawyers. I asked a friend who works in a different hospital to ask the risk managers who they would least like to come up against in a malpractice trial. With the pro bono lawyer by my side, I went to interview that firm. They took the case, warning me that the process would be long and painful. Was I up to it? I didn't know.

The firm filed the lawsuit, naming my husband and me as plaintiffs. Then began the excruciating experience of dealing with the hospital lawyers, their delaying tactics, and our depositions. Although my husband was able to participate in the depositions, I never knew exactly what he would say because of his brain injury. This made the process even more anxiety-provoking.

Through their deposition questions and discussions with our lawyers, the hospital attorneys intimated that my husband was a reckless driver (even though several other major accidents, including a fatality, had occurred that morning on the same stretch of road). They focused on his brain damage, suggesting that the loss of an arm didn't make much difference. They asked questions about our sexual compatibility, marital disagreements, and personal histories. If doctors think trial lawyers are sleazy, they have only to look to their own advocates for evidence of ugly behavior.

Months and months, and then a year, then two, passed. No settlement offers. I believe that the hospital lawyers were waiting for my husband to die, reducing the hospital's liability. At last the judge ordered the doctors' depositions to begin. And on the day before the first deposition (at which the extent and egregiousness of the errors would finally go on record), the hospital lawyers made an offer. Our lawyers said that it was fair, and I immediately accepted. It was finally over, or so I thought. But it is not over and never will be. Money, essential as it is, does not by itself right a wrong.

Disclosure and Closure

Pain and suffering are real, not just legal fictions. Even after years of therapy I still have nightmares involving loss of body parts. My husband has adjusted better than I have, partly because he has no memory of the events. My grandchildren are now old enough to ask about Grandpa's missing arm. Where is it? I do not want them to know just yet that doctors can make mistakes, so I say that the loss was part of the accident that put him in a wheelchair.

At present, persons who have suffered medical harm have only one channel of recourse—the tort system. Lawyers take cases on contingency, and their fees come out of an eventual award, if there is one. This system worked for me. Even so, the lack of a long-term care system that can manage complex cases like my husband's meant that the award provided only the minimum financial resources to allow me to cobble together a workable, though fragile, home care system. (My only alternative to suing the hospital was impoverishment so that my husband would be eligible for Medicaid. This would have ended my career and reduced the quality of our lives enormously.) But how many people can't get lawyers to take their cases because attorneys feel that the evidence is too weak, the odds of recovery too low, or the recoverable amount doesn't justify the huge cost of going to trial or reaching a settlement? How many families give up because they can't stand the strain?

Beyond whatever tort reforms may be advisable, some kind of nonadversarial system should exist for people who have suffered financially from medical error. Some potential models are the federal no-fault schemes for children who have experienced serious side effects from vaccines, or the federal compensation system for September 11 families. For some people, the benefits of certainty and speed may outweigh the downside of potentially lower compensation levels.

But even for people like me who do manage to receive compensation for medical error, money is only part of the solution. Lawsuits are filed not just for financial reasons but because people feel abandoned and aggrieved in ways that better communication and acknowledgment might alleviate. Doctors and risk managers underestimate both the importance that families place on knowing what happened to loved ones and the frustration they feel when stonewalled. If there were more openness, including apologies, some lawsuits might be forestalled and others settled quickly, without so much emotional toll on families and physicians. Our lawyers have reconstructed a fairly good but still incomplete picture of what happened to my husband; to this day we do not know the details.

Equally important, I have no idea what happened as a result of the inevitable hospital and, I assume, regulatory review. Good reasons exist to keep confidential a hospital's deliberations during a morbidity and mortality review, but I believe that it's essential to let patients and families know what measures have been taken to prevent a similar error.

Despite this experience, I have entrusted my husband's care to the same hospital and even on one occasion to the same ICU, where the care was excellent. But when he or anyone else in my family is hospitalized, I am constantly vigilant, mindful of how little it takes to turn routine into disaster.

⌁ Incidental Illness

*Working outside an academic medical setting shakes up
the assumptions of a newly minted doctor.*

Danielle Ofri

I t took several weeks after residency had ended for my body to recover.
And it took even longer for my mind. I couldn't quite believe that I would
never again spend another night in a hospital. Never again find myself
wandering deserted hallways at 3 a.m. Never sweat over another IV in a
veinless drug user. Never have to sleep in used sheets, shivering for lack of
a blanket. And I would never again have to introduce myself as a doctor-
in-training. I was finally a real doctor, whatever that meant.

Unable to decide whether to pursue a specialty fellowship in cardiology
or nephrology, I decided to do some temp work. I hooked up with a *locum
tenens* agency that was able to provide short-term assignments around the
country, usually filling in at short-staffed practices until full-time doctors
could be hired. My plan was to work for a month and then travel for as long
as the money would last, then work again. But I had to work first in order to
start the cycle. I quickly discovered that the academic medical cocoon in
which I was hatched did not, by any means, represent the way most people
received their health care. Most people saw their doctors in small offices or
community-based clinics. They rarely set foot inside a huge tertiary care hospital like the one in New York where I'd trained. Most doctors practiced in
small groups, without the benefit of twenty-four-hour availability of hema-
tologists, pulmonologists, and cardiovascular surgeons.

There were other, more subtle differences. How, for example, in this quiet
world of outpatient medicine, does one know when a life is saved? In residency training, saving a life was always dramatic. It was a uniquely physical
and sensory experience: pounding the chest and shocking the heart, scram-

Volume 23, Number 4: 197–201. July/August 2004.

bling for a pulse, smelling the singed flesh, cringing at the violent intubation and inelegant intravenous lines. The perspiration built beneath poly-
ester scrubs as the brain battled to think clearly amid competing shouts and
jostling bodies and bloody gauze. There were no subtleties to confound;
everyone knew when a life was saved or lost.

In the outpatient setting it wasn't clear when I was having any effect on
someone's life, let alone saving it. I found myself sifting through a morass of
vague, unrelated complaints, wondering, "Is this the symptom that really
means something?" There was no overhead operator paging me to an emergency, *stat*, and no dramatic restoration of the heartbeat informing me that
my task was accomplished.

Unnecessary Testing

On my second day in a clinic in northwestern New Mexico, a nurse handed
me a chart. A patient was seeking referral to a psychiatrist, and the clinic required a standard panel of blood tests before any referral. Normally the nurse
would relay the results, but the computer had flagged one value as "abnormal." By protocol, the chart had to be reviewed by a physician. I happened
to be standing around sipping tea, so I was drafted.

The academic physicians from my residency program disapproved of routine blood tests on healthy patients. They insisted on scientific documentation of the risk–benefit ratio of each and every test, disparaging physicians
"out in the community" who weren't up to date on the latest research and
couldn't cite the tenets of "evidence-based medicine."

I launched into a tirade to all who cared to listen. "There is no hard evidence," I exhorted, "for this kind of testing." I waved the lab sheet dramatically in the air. "This is a perfect example of unnecessary testing that could
lead to more harm than good for the patient." Eager to flex my scholarship,
still gleaming from residency, and having just taken my medical boards, I argued that the vast majority of abnormal lab results in healthy people were
clinically inconsequential. They would necessitate costly and risky additional tests but would most likely turn out to be "false positives." But preach
as I might about the theoretical risks of routine testing, a human being still
waited in my office for the results.

Paul Davis (not his real name) was a fifty-six-year-old white man who had
recently retired from his job as a machinist. He had worked in an asbestos-

laden environment, giving up cigarettes only after a coworker succumbed to lung cancer. He had no medical history and continued to lead a physically active life. His main complaint was intermittent depression. One of his children had been killed in a car accident a few years back. Each year, as the anniversary approached, he found himself unable to sleep, plagued by nightmares and feelings of hopelessness. He was cognizant of the pattern and would routinely seek professional help, going into therapy and taking antidepressant medications until the symptoms abated.

On the lab sheet Mr. Davis's iron level was mildly elevated. If clinic protocol didn't require me to discuss this with him, I might have ignored it as a false positive because he was so healthy and had no family history of medical problems. Earlier I had commented sarcastically to my colleagues, "What's he going to have, hemochromatosis or something? He'll probably die of lung cancer from cigarettes and asbestos before anything else gets him."

I sat opposite Mr. Davis in the tiny examining room. His rough-hewn features reflected a lifetime of physical labor. His hands were too big for his body, and he shuffled them awkwardly. Attentive green eyes flickered behind several days of beard growth. I told him that I didn't think the iron level was significant, but because of the clinic protocol I would have to do another few blood tests.

Being Wrong

I drove home grumbling to myself about the lack of academic standards in the community. The air was stiflingly dusty, and I was forced to keep my windows closed. In the back seat of my rental car I stored both t-shirts and heavy sweaters to keep up with the blistering hot days and the chilly nights. The town was located near the 300,000-acre Navajo reservation, and the clinic was frequented by a mix of Navajos, Hispanics, and Anglos, united by their lack of private health insurance. The clinic itself was tagged onto a strip mall, tucked away at the far end of a vast parking lot behind a low-end department store.

I drove through the shabby downtown toward my hotel. The squat buildings had turquoise trim on adobe-colored brick. They could almost be quaint but looked too wearied from suburban onslaught. The pawnshops and mobile home dealerships that lined the main road were shadowed by starkly majestic slabs of ochre granite. I stopped at the public library to read the Sunday *New York Times* — my weekly dose of civilization, even if it didn't arrive until the following Wednesday.

The next day Mr. Davis's lab results clearly indicated hemochromatosis, a serious metabolic disorder of relentless iron deposition in the body's vital organs. My jaw froze, and my heart sank as the numbers on the page metamorphosed into the clinical reality of liver disease and heart failure. Shame crept over me. How could I have been so cavalier and so utterly wrong? I had just taken the boards, hadn't I? I was even more horrified to note a flicker of pride beneath the shame, a carnal spark of bravado at making such an "interesting" diagnosis. I mean, it wasn't every day that a rare metabolic disorder was diagnosed in a general medical clinic — the kind you had to look up in the textbooks to remember the details. Even through all my years in residency, I'd never diagnosed hemochromatosis.

My clinic colleagues were congratulating me. In a world of common colds and stomachaches, hemochromatosis was downright exciting. "You just saved his life," they said. "What a lucky man!" Lucky? I wasn't so sure. I had to tell this man sitting before me that although he felt healthy, he in fact had a genetic disease that was potentially fatal. Every organ of his body could be destroyed by the iron. The liver was at particular risk. He required immediate treatment and a needle biopsy of the liver. His siblings and children needed urgently to be tested.

Delivering Bad News

Mr. Davis looked intently at me with a trusting, almost innocent, expression. The fine bristles of his unshaven beard framed his face with a shadow so that only his green eyes stood out. They didn't blink much or flicker; they just rested on my gaze. And then he uttered those awful words: "Are you sure, doctor?" I drew in a painful breath. Sure? What does it mean to be sure? My mind raced, checking and rechecking the facts, scouring the corners, chasing the doubts. When had I heard that lecture in med school? Where was that part on the boards? Sure? What a rotten word. What an insidious concept. No one can ever be sure about anything. Wasn't that Heisenburg's Principle of Uncertainty? Who ever condescended to invent such a word anyway? What was it doing in our lexicon? Deceitful bearer of false security — it ought to be banished from the dictionaries. It didn't deserve to be roving the

English language with all the other honest, well-meaning words. "Yes," I squeezed out. "I am sure." Mr. Davis nodded. I braced myself for the instinctive panic and the flood of anger or fear or bewilderment, but he was quiet. His eyes continued their even gaze, his lids remained calm. His hands shuffled between themselves as they had been doing all along. And now he was nodding with a gentle periodicity.

Speak, my mind demanded. Say something. React. Get angry at me. But Mr. Davis stayed as he was, eyes gazing, head nodding, hands shuffling. My own discomfort bubbled over, and I burst in with unbidden answers. "The iron builds up in your body, you see. We don't exactly know why, but you absorb more iron than most people. When people are severely low in iron, we give them blood. In your case we do the opposite; we take away blood. It can slow the progression of the disease."

"When would you do that?" Mr. Davis asked soberly. "Today," I swallowed dryly. "Now." Mr. Davis continued to nod. "And," I added, "we have to check your liver. That's usually the first organ to be affected. A needle biopsy will tell us what stage the disease is at." Mr. Davis was quiet and almost complacent. Gazing, nodding, shuffling. Why wasn't he angry at me for my falsely reassuring words yesterday? Why wasn't he angry at this horrible disease that could eat away at his body? Maybe, I wondered, a strange disease with a big, fancy name and lots of treatments was trivial after the loss of a child. Maybe his body had already been eaten away by grief, and there wasn't much left for the hemochromatosis.

I watched Mr. Davis in his suspended state. Did I really save his life? Perhaps, but I didn't feel the elation of success. If I had applied the rigorous scientific beliefs of my academic training, he never would have been tested, and his illness would not have been detected at such an early stage. More than that, though, a healthy man had just been sentenced to a life of illness. How could I rejoice at that? Physically, his body was no different than it was ten minutes ago, but now he was a man with a "problem." His medical records would henceforth commence with the weighted words, "a fifty-six-year-old white man with hemochromatosis . . ."

So many decisions in his life—medical, financial, social—would now have to pass the litmus test: But what about the hemochromatosis? Could this sinus medicine now hurt me? Can I eat raw seafood? Travel? Play sports? Buy life insurance? What if I want to apply for a job? With all these medical expenses, can we afford a vacation this year? Should I tell my friends? Mr.

Davis had no symptoms with which to verify his brand-new illness, nor had he any medical knowledge with which to understand it. He had to believe a handful of words from an out-of-town doctor whom he'd never met before.

I carefully printed the word "hemochromatosis" on a slip of paper while the nurse prepared Mr. Davis for his first phlebotomy treatment. As his iron-laden blood dripped slowly into the bag, I was overwhelmed by the quiet drama unfolding around me. It wasn't like a code in the hospital, but the intensity was unmistakable. It reminded me of watching a great dancer, in whom a subtle gesture, with the right music, could deliver as much emotional impact as a troupe of whirling, leaping acrobats.

I said goodbye to Mr. Davis after his treatment. He was about twenty feet down the hallway when he turned and called out to me, "Hey, doc, what about my depression? Will I still get my medications? Can I still see the psychiatrist?" I froze in my tracks, my skin bristling. I had completely forgotten the reason he had come to the clinic. In all of the tumult surrounding his new asymptomatic illness, I had lost sight of the problem that was really giving him symptoms. I quickly reassured him that he would get his referral to the psychiatrist, noting bitterly to myself that I had provided him with far more fodder for discussion than he had likely anticipated. I grabbed a prescription pad and fished in my pocket for a pen. I started to scribble down the prescription for his antidepressant, but my hand halted in midsentence. What about the hemochromatosis, I thought, a chill running along my fingers? Would I make things worse? Could this medicine interfere with the hemochromatosis? I didn't want to get myself in any trouble; what would someone say if they saw I'd added extra medications just when this disease was diagnosed? Maybe I should hold off on any new medicines until we knew what stage his disease is at—the less complicating factors the better.

Complicating factors? The pen nearly slipped from my grip. What could be more complicating than the depression associated with the death of a child? How could I even consider not giving him this prescription? I caught my sliding pen. I scratched the ink deep into the pad to make sure it was legible and permanent. I signed my name at the bottom, then stopped to catch my breath. I'd obviously want to pick the antidepressant with the least interactions with the liver, but the fact that my instinct had been to avoid it altogether, and more for my piece of mind than anything else, gave me the shivers. I'd almost committed malpractice—moral malpractice. I'd almost withheld this medicine he needed so desperately.

⌢ The Rest Is Silence

Hospitals and doctors should beware of what can fill the space of their silence after a loved one's death.

MICHAEL ROWE

Jesse, my nineteen-year-old son, had been shivering constantly for the past twenty-four hours, and now his lips were shivering too. We stood around the bed, his mother, his stepmother, and I. Terri, his nurse, was in and out of the room hanging blood, platelets, and fresh frozen plasma on one of the poles at the corners of his bed. It had been a night and a day and a night since his last downturn. The three of us had gone without sleep, nodding off as we warmed bags of blood against our bodies before passing them to the nurses to be hung before the last bag was empty. The nurses said that doing this would make it easier for Jesse as the blood went through his IVs.

The first downturn had come three months ago, when Jesse's surgeons took him back to the operating room four days after his liver transplant because his temperature had gone up and he needed more and more Fentanyl for the pain in his belly. (Jesse needed the transplant because of cirrhosis of the liver, which had been diagnosed two years earlier, shortly before his surgery for ulcerative colitis—an intestinal disorder that is associated with developing liver disease.) They discovered that while connecting the hepatic artery of his new liver to his intestine, they had inadvertently caused an intestinal perforation during the difficult task of cutting through the intestinal adhesions that had formed after Jesse's surgery for ulcerative colitis. That perforation led to peritonitis, and peritonitis led to sepsis. Less than three weeks after his transplant Dr. Dorand, the attending surgeon, told us that Jesse had only one to two days to live. But Jesse rallied and received a second transplant. Before this last bout with sepsis there had been another perforation—this time caused by Jesse's weakened state and poor nutrition—then another

Volume 21, Number 4: 232–236. July/August 2002.

bout of sepsis that ruined his second new liver, another "one-to-two-days to live" speech, and another rally leading to plans for a third transplant.

I felt the bed rail sink a little to my left. It was Dr. Dorand. My wife, Gail, suggested that we all go outside the room to talk.

Dr. Dorand stood at the far end of the nurse's station. Dr. Broward, the nephrologist supervising attempts to give Jesse the dialysis he needed to clear toxins from his blood, stood at his side. The ICU attending physician, the residents, the nurses, and we stood around them. We talked about what to do.

"We could take him back into surgery to look for a discrete source of bleeding," said Dr. Dorand. "I'm a surgeon, so that's my impulse. I want to do something. If I did it, it would be with some hope." He paused. It was clear that he'd have a hard time mustering any hope for Jesse now.

"If he were your child, what would you do?" I asked.

There was silence. I wondered if my question was in poor taste but then thought, no, Dr. Dorand would understand that I had to ask it. He stood mute for what seemed like several minutes, looking around, not at the others as though to be rescued, but behind them. I wondered if I should break the silence by rephrasing the question, but something told me not to. Finally he looked at me.

"I would wait. I think it's more likely that the surgery would kill him than help him. I would wait for an opening."

Dr. Broward agreed. He couldn't give Jesse his daily dialysis because when they started the dialysis machine his blood pressure would plummet. "The best thing to do now is to wait and see if we can find an opening to take action. If Jesse's blood pressure stabilizes, then we can look for another opening from there."

The three of us—Gail, Rachel (Jesse's mother), and I—looked at one another and agreed. An hour from now there might be another decision to make, but for now we would wait. The meeting broke up, and Dr. Dorand left for surgery. I told Gail I had to go lie down in our favorite resting place.

I don't know if I slept or not, so I must have. I heard Gail's voice. "Michael? I think you'd better come down to the room."

We stood outside Jesse's room and looked back and forth from him to the blood pressure monitor above his bed. Minutes later it was over. Dr. Rivera, the ICU attending physician, called an end to the code, and everyone was out of the room in a blur. Terri, who had been counting the beats for Dr. Rivera, brushed by us on her way out and let out a great sob.

We took photos and cards off the wall. People came and went. The attending gastroenterologist asked if we wanted an autopsy. If not, they could remove Jesse's tubes and IVs. If so, they would have to leave them in until the autopsy was performed. No, we didn't want an autopsy. Jesse's body had been battered and beaten, poked and prodded enough. The transplant coordinator told us that there would be no autopsy and that the body would be kept at the hospital morgue until our funeral director picked it up. I kept wondering if Dr. Dorand would come back. Gail's sister arrived to take us back home.

From Trust to Mistrust

Rachel and I decided to have Jesse cremated and made separate funeral arrangements in our separate hometowns. I waited for Dr. Dorand's call. The power of newborn grief had blinded me to the fact that it might be hard for a surgeon to have an ongoing relationship with the father of the boy who had died on his watch. Perhaps I felt close to Dr. Dorand because he had reached out to Jesse a few weeks before his transplant, telling him that he had his whole life ahead of him, while reminding him of the risks. Perhaps it was because a few weeks before Jesse's last downturn, Dr. Dorand had played guitar and sung "Here Comes the Sun" for him, at the risk of ridicule from his colleagues. And there were tears in his eyes when I asked him what he would do if Jesse were his son.

Two days before the funeral I got a call from my funeral director, who informed me that upon arriving at the hospital to pick up Jesse's body, he was told that it had been taken to the city medical examiner's office for a full autopsy and that Rachel or I would have to come to the city morgue to identify Jesse before that office would release his body. I called Jill, the liver transplant coordinator. Her quick action straightened it out—no autopsy was performed, and the body was released to our funeral director. But I asked for an investigation of how communication between the ICU and the hospital morgue could have broken down so badly. The explanation, which blamed our funeral director, was preposterous and, it seemed to me, designed to protect the hospital against a lawsuit. I was angry and amazed that anyone could think we would fall for this inaccurate accounting.

Over the next few weeks I came to realize that Dr. Dorand was not going to call. I also began to receive the first of what would be dozens of letters from the hospital, mostly bills, from the many consulting specialists. These came from the ICU and nearly every hospital department, even though my health plan had negotiated a "global price" to cover all expenses. One bill was addressed to Ms. Jessie Harlan-Rowe. Another, for $357,000, offered me the option of using my MasterCard.

I wrote a letter to the liver team about our feelings. Dr. Dorand called and invited us to meet with him about setting up a physician-survivor group to develop standards for how the team would deal with death. Gail and I met with him and agreed to help, but weeks passed and we heard nothing. I wrote again, this time to the director of the hospital, listing our grievances. I received a letter informing me that the hospital was looking into things and would get back to me. No one did.

By this time I was beginning to wonder if lack of empathy was the problem, after all. What if Dr. Dorand and the others didn't want to talk to us because they had made mistakes that had cost Jesse his life? What if the perforation that occurred during Jesse's first liver transplant was not a "surgical accident," as Dr. Dorand had described it, but a surgical error? Should they have suspected, much earlier than they did, that his belly was filling up with intestinal contents? In the silence that followed my son's death, trust died and mistrust took its place.

One morning, about three months after Jesse's death, Gail and I sat at the kitchen table and talked over breakfast. "We want to be paid," she said. "And if we can't have Jesse back we want to be paid in understanding, and if we can't have understanding then we want to be paid in money."

Slippery Slope to a Lawsuit

I followed the green stripe painted at a three-foot height on the tunnel wall in the hospital basement until I reached the medical records office. A Mrs. Lopez introduced herself and led me through another set of tunnels formed by banks of five-drawer metal file cabinets on either side. I sat at a Formica-top desk. She brought out volume after thick volume of Jesse's chart, seven volumes in all. I started at volume one and studied nurses' and doctors' notes and surgical and lab reports. There was no smoking gun here, but I found reason to think that Jesse's doctors should have diagnosed a perforation and gotten him back into surgery long before they did. I had Mrs. Lopez copy some pages for me and went home.

Over the next nine months I reviewed the chart material with a neighbor who is an ICU nurse; through a friend I contacted a physician who found things that disturbed him and who then tried to get a liver specialist to look at the chart. I phoned and wrote to the hospital asking for missing lab reports and x-rays. I talked to several malpractice attorneys before finding one who was willing to talk to a doctor about Jesse's case, assuming I could find one. Finally, nine months after my visit to the medical records office, I found a liver specialist who told me I had cause but that Jesse's was not an obvious and flagrant case of malpractice and might be difficult to prove. This doctor talked to my attorney the next day, and the attorney declined to take the case. My investigation had ended.

I finally did hear from Dr. Dorand again, around the time I spoke with the attorney. It turned out that he was calling a physician-survivor meeting after all, and had done some work on a policy for the liver team to follow up with family members after a patient's death. The meeting came too late for us, and I don't know what the outcome was, although I'm glad it was going to take place.

It has been six years since Jesse died. The people I work for in New Haven—those who are homeless, are mentally ill, have a drug addiction, or live with their children in public housing projects where the street lights get shot out to give cover of darkness for nighttime drug dealing—endure daily traumas that, I expect, will never be my family's lot. I am aware, too, that a certain privilege surrounds being the father of a child who died from a liver transplant—that of having a job that provides the insurance to pay for the surgery and that scarce organ in the first place. Still, the death of a child, or any loved one, is a grievous thing. That event was made worse for us by silence from the only people we thought were in a position to understand what we had gone through.

I dealt with all of this in various ways—by writing about Jesse, by having the good fortune not to be biologically prone to deep depression, and by a learned capacity to control my rage. Jim, a fellow parent whose baby daughter had died of biliary atresia (a condition in which the bile ducts fail to develop as they should) knocked over a newspaper stand outside the hospital and would have been arrested if his wife hadn't been there to explain his behavior to the police. Despite our warnings that it would be stolen (and it was), my mother placed a stone with Jesse's name on it under a tree she'd had planted for him in a park in Canada, the country of his dreams, although he never went there.

Jim, my mother, and many of those who sue doctors, as well as many of those who do not, have no place else to hang their grief when that grief—and seemingly their loved one's life—is being ignored, even declared, in the space left by silence, a thing of no value. I too felt this, even though the rational side of me knew that the hospital and doctors did not intend to show us such extreme disrespect.

It is not that people sue without medical cause, but that they sue, in part, because they have no place else to go for recognition (from those who should be among the first to give it) that their loved one's life and their loss matter. My wife's comment about "being paid" came at a time when we still didn't know whether we were reacting to lack of empathy or lack of good medical care. The notion of payment may seem crude when talking about human life, but the term is correct: When trust exits, debits and credits enter the vacuum that nature abhors. Trust gives passage over doubt, disbelief, and dark possibilities, and its absence nurtures those same qualities. And while I've made this point in relation to lawsuits and the contemplation of lawsuits, surely it applies to other aspects of the doctor-caretaker relationship after a patient's death. Death is a failure when the aim was greater health, but with a little bit of effort it need not be only a failure. Both doctors and family members might benefit from words and actions that bridge the silence that death leaves behind.

∽ DNAbling Parents

Genetics technology brings both hope and excruciating personal decisions to patients who use it.

LISA SWEETINGHAM

On a Sunday morning in late November 2000, Karen McGuire went to Mass with a special request for God. As she walked up the aisle to take Holy Communion, she thought about her secret—a recent home pregnancy test had confirmed that she was pregnant. As the priest placed the wafer on her tongue, she swallowed it and prayed that her developing baby would grow up healthy and strong.

A month later the thirty-seven-year-old human resources manager and

Volume 22, Number 5: 172–176. September/October 2003.

her husband, Gerry, thirty-four, a graduate student in history, traveled from their Long Island apartment to Karen's brother's house in Boston. At bedtime she followed her thirty-six-year-old brother Scott as he powered himself by electric wheelchair into his room. She helped him to the bed, undressed him, and followed him into the bathroom where she laid him back into the shower on a reclining seat made of netting and plastic pipes. She bathed him, washed his hair twice (how he likes it), brushed his teeth, and helped him back to bed. As she placed pillows behind his neck and set up the ventilator that helps him breathe at night, she looked lovingly into the eyes of the man who had once been the little boy she helped raise. And she hoped and prayed that the child growing inside her would not share his affliction—Duchenne's muscular dystrophy (DMD).

DMD occurs in about one of every 3,500 boys born worldwide, causing increased muscle weakness as their bodies grow. Until they hit kindergarten, there's usually no indication that anything is wrong. Survival is rare beyond the late twenties. Pneumonia or a stopped heart are the two most common ways that someone with muscular dystrophy dies. There is no cure.

Technology and Hope

Karen and Gerry shared with me the story of their quest for a healthy baby when I was a journalism student at Columbia University working on an article about assisted reproductive technology. When I first met the McGuires, they had already spent two years and more than $20,000 on preimplantation genetic diagnosis, or PGD, in an attempt to guarantee that their first child would be healthy. If that attempt had worked (it did not—in the end, Karen's pregnancy was accomplished without technology), the McGuire baby would have joined an estimated 1,000 PGD infants born worldwide since 1989, according to the Genetics and Public Policy Center. The process, which is not as simple as it sounds, begins with in vitro fertilization (IVF). When each blastocyst is about eight cells old, a single cell is tested for the specific genetic mutation that one or both partners may carry. Only those testing negative are transferred to the mother's womb. Nine months later, if all else goes well, a healthy baby is born. Testing is available for more than fifty genetic disorders including Tay-Sachs, cystic fibrosis, Huntington's, and hemophilia. PGD's use is increasing steadily among parents who want to ensure that their lethal genes will not be passed on.

I was trained to approach all issues with fairness and skepticism, and the morality of choices that PGD permits gave me plenty to be skeptical about. I pictured the day when ambitious parents could drop into their doctor's office and choose a tall, perfectly formed baby boy with a chart-popping IQ. While I dug deeper into the science and ethics behind PGD, Karen's story of two failed PGD attempts followed by a jittery natural pregnancy unfolded before me. Her experience reveals what life was like before PGD for couples with familial genetic disorders who must endure ten to fifteen weeks of high anxiety as they wait for a chorionic villus sampling (CVS) or amniocentesis result. If tests determine that their baby has the family disease, they are forced to consider having a very sick child or a second-trimester abortion. In fact, from my interviews with genetic counselors and physicians, I learned that many parents turn to PGD in terrible grief only after the loss of a first child from a disease they didn't even know was in their genes.

I spent almost six months interviewing the McGuires. Karen said she hoped that by sharing her experience with me, others would understand what an arduous process PGD is. She wants people to know that it is filled with failures and physical trials that make it a highly undesirable route for healthy parents who simply want to "design a baby." I also began to think more about my own extended family's genetic history. No fatal childhood diseases plague our brood, but there's a raging predisposition toward alcoholism and depression in both sets of grandparents that skipped over me and my brothers but has rendered a number of aunts and uncles in perpetual states of self-destruction. If genetic markers for these ills could be tested for one day, would I attempt to save my own children from such hardship? Despite the intrinsic environmental influences on diseases such as alcoholism and mental illness, I am certain that advances in human genome research will deliver the keys to unlock many of the mysteries of human nature. Personally, when it comes to nonfatal traits, I prefer the mystery. But witnessing the McGuires' ordeal has made me keenly aware of PGD's value for eliminating fatal genetic disease, which far outweighs the technology's potential for misuse.

Mission: Healthy Baby

Karen's reasons for trying technology to better her chances of having a healthy baby were rooted in her childhood. When she was twelve years old, her doctors warned her that one day having kids of her own would be like playing Russian roulette. As a DMD carrier, she has a 50 percent chance of giving the disease to a son and of passing the carrier trait to a daughter. Still, she said, by her mid-thirties, with babies on the brain, her first impulse was to think, "I have good luck, my husband has good luck, we'll be okay." But Gerry wasn't satisfied with their odds and didn't want to have to face the abortion question should their dare with nature backfire. "My Catholicism was kicking in, and I felt guilty," he said. "I saw what Karen's brother goes through just to breathe, and I saw Karen having to live with that her whole life. I couldn't imagine having to watch my own kid go through the same thing." The McGuires also decided against adoption and agreed that PGD seemed like their best hope for a healthy family.

In fall 1999 Karen had her first appointment with a specialist in infertility and reproductive surgery at Cornell University's Weill Medical College in New York City. Here she learned the basics: One try at a healthy baby would include a series of drug cycles (about $5,000) prior to egg retrieval surgery ($8,900), PGD testing (free at the time because it was covered by an experimental research protocol, but most centers charge between $1,000 and $5,000), then transfer of the preselected blastocysts. Karen also learned that her odds of conception were about 46 percent.

Over the next few weeks Karen's body was prepped for egg retrieval. Doctors took blood samples, x-rayed her fallopian tubes, and prescribed drugs to induce maximum egg production. Gerry learned how to give Karen daily injections of these "psycho drugs," as he affectionately called them, which wreaked havoc with her hormones, making her feel irritable and out of control. "The process really consumes your whole life," she recalled. "You can't go anywhere because you have to plan to be home for your shots." Karen also began to obsess over her late childbearing age of thirty-seven and how it affected her odds of conception.

"Congratulations, you're pregnant," a Cornell nurse reported to Karen by phone in March 2000. A few days earlier, doctors had transferred two DMD-free embryos to Karen's womb. She was elated. "I got that first phone call, and I just didn't know any better," she said. What she didn't understand was that at this stage it was simply a chemical pregnancy in which her levels of HCG (human chorionic gonadotropin) had risen and all maternal signals were a "go," but the embryo had failed. Karen got her period soon after and was left with nothing. She wanted to try PGD again right away, but Gerry needed a break. So they waited until August to begin a second cycle of drugs, write a second batch of checks, and try IVF and PGD again. "It was going to be my thirty-seventh birthday in a couple of days," Karen said. "I was hoping this was gonna be my birthday present." Karen's birthday passed with no gift from modern medicine, barren as before.

Frustrated, the McGuires decided to bring the business of baby-making back into their bedroom, letting the genetic chips fall where they may. Their third attempt at conception—in their own home, unassisted, free of needles, drugs, and doctors—was a natural success but constituted a huge risk.

Big Gamble

Karen's pregnancy was a dream fulfilled, yet she anguished over the potential consequences of what she'd done. She agonized over the possibility of having an abortion if her fetus carried her brother's disease. At the same time, she was quietly angry with abortion critics who often stood next to her at church. "I just want to say to them, 'You've never walked in my shoes; you didn't help me raise my brother; you didn't have twenty years of nightmares about how your brother's going to die.'" She prayed for a healthy baby.

In February 2001, at nineteen weeks, amniocentesis revealed that she was carrying a boy—who had a fifty-fifty chance of developing DMD. "I could've walked out that day and begun enjoying the pregnancy if they'd told me it was a girl," she recalled. Karen's father, a senior technician at a genetics research lab in Massachusetts, had helped to create the test for the specific type of Duchenne's that the family carried (an endeavor inspired by his son's affliction). He was the one she trusted most to perform the next crucial step: DNA testing that would tell them definitively if her baby was affected.

Now their main unknown was the genetic mystery of the baby's DNA. Karen's father would shepherd the testing but wouldn't have an answer for two torturous weeks. To prepare for bad news, Karen asked her family doctor on Long Island about abortion options. He described a termination that could be scheduled on a day's notice. "That week was the worst," Karen said. "Gerry was in the middle of papers and tests. We'd come home at night and just look at each other and cry."

Meanwhile, her belly was growing, but the joys of motherhood eluded her. Her clothes no longer fit, so she went to the shopping mall. "I was so depressed," she said. "There was a motherhood store, but it didn't make sense for me to go in there yet." A friend who mourned the loss of her own aborted baby after learning that it would have had a fatal genetic disease advised Karen that naming it and having a funeral ultimately gave her closure. "She said her only regret was not having held it in her arms," Karen recalled. "She said, 'You're parents right now, and this will be the first decision as parents that you're making about your baby.'" When Karen came home with information on baby cemetery plots, Gerry said he didn't think he could go through with aborting, naming, and then burying their baby.

On a Friday in March, Karen went to church after work. "I didn't know how I was going to get through the weekend," she said. She found herself asking less that her baby be safe, and more "please help me to deal with whatever I'm gonna have to go through." At the same time, in a research lab in Boston, Karen's father was putting her baby's cells through a DNA-sequencing machine. He labeled his grandson's cells SM for "Shane, male." Karen had told him of her fondness for the Irish name Shane, which, she was told, in Hebrew means "gracious gift from God."

DNA sequencing on Shane's cells was complete at 4:30 a.m. on Saturday. Karen's father was so nervous about the results that he couldn't sleep. He drove back to the lab, bracing himself for the answer. "He called me at 7:30 a.m.; I didn't hear anything when I answered, and I thought it was a crank call," Karen said. "But then I heard him say my name, and I knew everything was OK." She reached over to Gerry, who was just waking, and sobbed, "Everything's OK." Her dad was crying on the other end of the phone. "He was so excited," she said. "He told me, 'I've been crying for fifteen minutes and had to pull myself together before I called.'"

Shane McGuire made a healthy arrival on July 24, 2001, at 5:16 a.m.—the same day as Gerry's father's birthday. "Gerry's dad passed away when Gerry was thirteen," Karen said. "No wonder Shane was so lucky; he's got a very special guardian angel." The McGuires would like to have another child, but they are no longer willing to rely on their luck and are certain they will give PGD another try.

Troubling Personal Choices

As the number and type of genetic tests available increase, more couples like the McGuires will turn to PGD to eliminate genetic diseases. The McGuires discovered that PGD may hold great promise, but it is not simple, nor is its success guaranteed. A new future through genetic technology is still an uncertain, expensive, and emotionally and physically draining roller coaster ride. Ability to pay for procedures can be a formidable obstacle for many: Karen and Gerry handed over their life savings—money intended for a down payment on a first home—to cover the cost of two attempts at IVF and PGD. But beyond cost, in this brave new age of genetic technology, people who use it must be willing to accept the pitfalls and failures ahead and to face the consequences of decisions made during very trying times.

My skepticism about PGD still lingers. The technique is ethically troubling. I am uneasy about its nontherapeutic uses such as for sex selection by healthy couples. I am hopeful that some parents, if well informed, will decide against PGD should their alternatives seem less daunting. However, having observed the McGuires' experience up close, I believe that decisions about whether to use PGD belong only to the people involved. As Karen said, "Someone at work told Gerry, 'What's the big deal? Karen's taken care of a handicapped kid before, she can do it again.' It makes me crazy. How dare someone presume what it's like for us?"

⌣ What Are We Going to Do with Dad?

A geriatrician stands by during his father's downward spiral into old age, disability, and dementia.

JERALD WINAKUR

My father is eighty-six years old. He was never a big man, except perhaps to me when I was his little boy. At most he was five feet, eight inches tall and weighed 160 pounds. Today he weighs barely 120. Maybe he is five feet two. He teeters on spindly legs, a parched blade of grass in the wind, refusing the walker his doctor recommends or the arm extended in support by those of us who love him. He doesn't know what day it is. He sleeps most of the time, barely eats. Shaving exhausts him. His clothes hang like a scarecrow's. Getting him in for a haircut is a major ordeal. He is very

Volume 24, Number 4: 1064–1072. July/August 2005.

deaf but won't wear his hearing aids or loses them as often as a kid might misplace his marbles. He drives my mother—five years younger—crazy to tears.

My only sibling, the architect, asks me every time we are together (which is often because we all live in the same town) and every time we speak on the phone (which is almost every day because we are a close family now in crisis): "What are we going to do with Dad?" As if there must be a definitive answer, some fix—say, putting a grab bar in the bathroom or increasing the width of the doorways. Something that is according to code.

He asks me this question not only out of fear and frustration, not only out of a realization that it is time for the adult children of a progressively dementing elderly parent to act, but also because he figures that his older brother, who has been practicing medicine for almost thirty years, should know the answer. I do not know the answer. I do not have a pat solution for my father or yours—neither as a son, a man past middle age with grown children of his own; nor as a doctor, a specialist in geriatrics, and a credentialed long-term care medical director.

In the United States today there are thirty-five million geriatric patients— over age sixty-five—and of these, 4.5 million are over age eighty-five, now characterized as the "old old." The American Medical Directors Association, the professional organization that credentials physicians in long-term care, has certified only 1,900 doctors in the entire country. As we baby boomers go about our lives, frozen into our routines of work and family responsibilities, a vast inland sea of elders is building. By 2020 it is projected that there will be fifty-three million Americans over age sixty-five, 6.5 million of whom will be "old old." Many of you will be among them. America will be inundated with old folks, each with a unique set of circumstances: medical history and the manifestations of the particular dementing process; medication use; emotional and psychological makeup, including past traumas and present-day fears; family dynamics; support structures; and finances.

Compounding all of this is the sad and frustrating fact that our government appears to have no policy vision for long-term elder care. Our leaders seem to wish—perhaps reflecting our own collective yearnings as a vain, youth-worshipping society—that when the time comes, the elderly will take their shuffling tired selves, their drooling and incontinence, their demented ravings, their drain on family and national resources, and sprawl out on an ice floe to be carried off to a white, comforting place, never to be heard from again.

The Role of the Skilled Nursing Unit

For the past nine years I have been the medical director of my hospital's skilled nursing unit, or SNU, as we call it. This unit receives transfers from all areas of the acute care hospital when attending physicians feel that their patients have reached a point where they no longer need acute care services yet are unable to return home. Sometimes it is obvious what we have to do: finish out a course of intravenous antibiotics in a patient with an infected wound or provide a few more days of rehab to a competent elder who has just undergone a hip replacement. But more and more, as our patients grow older and more frail, it becomes clear that the attending physicians have requested that their patients come to the SNU because they don't know what else to do with them.

Each week I attend the SNU team care conference. Every staff professional who has a role in caring for patients on the unit attends, so around the tables pushed together in the unit's "activity room," amid the puzzles and games almost none of the patients have the ability to play, the magazines most no longer have the eyesight or insight to read, sit a registered nurse; geriatric nurse specialist; pharmacist; social worker; activity coordinator; physical, occupational, speech, and respiratory therapists; dietitian; and myself. We discuss each patient in turn and review each medication list. The nurses provide up-to-the-minute reports on medical progress or setbacks; the therapists discuss the rehabilitation status and whether the patient is proceeding toward goals set the previous week; the patient's weight and diet are reviewed; we hear about the situation at home, the help or lack thereof that we can expect from family or other caretakers, and the patient's insurance and what it may or may not provide. Our main goal is to answer one major question: What are we going to do with this patient? Where can we safely send him—given his medical, social, and financial circumstances—and expect him to maintain his highest level of functioning, his remaining dignity? Very often, we don't know.

After we review each patient's case, families are encouraged to attend. Most do not—often, I think, because they are afraid we will tell them there is nothing more we can do. And they are already despondent, overwhelmed by Dad's downhill progress and the acute event that brought him to the hospital (the pneumonia, the fall, the stroke), bewildered by his deteriorating course (the mental confusion, the weakness) while there, and angered and frustrated in dealing with the bureaucracy (callous nurses, inattentive aides). Even with the attending physicians, who often drift quickly in and out on their rounds like white-coated apparitions.

So now your dad's physician—maybe the one person you thought could solve all of this, the one person you trusted (although less and less so in these days of "managed care," because it is hard to trust someone you might have just met or whose name was picked at random from a list of random names)—comes into his room and says, "I don't think there is much more we can do for him here." Your mind reels. Nothing more to do? In America? Home of the most advanced health care in the world? The land of Medicare and WebMD? You think about all the glowing seniors—continent, smiling, sexually active—in those drug ads on TV, or the aging but robust movie stars on the cover of the AARP magazine. Nothing to do?! What, I'm supposed to take him home like this? You gotta be kidding, doc! And anyway, he was just fine until he came to the hospital!

The doctor sighs. She has been through this many times and still doesn't quite know how to handle it. Even though the ravages of aging are not her fault, she feels the stern gaze of Hippocrates on her back and wants to do more. She might remind you—tactfully—that this patient, your father, lying with sallow distorted face, partial paralysis, a Foley catheter now hanging out of his penis attached to a bag clipped to the bedrail, was not fine when he came to the hospital. He was not shanghaied from his home where he sat smoking his pipe and reading the *Wall Street Journal*. Rather, this man, her patient whom she doesn't know what to do with at this moment, arrived in the ER at 4 a.m. hypertensive and gurgling, brought in by ambulance after he passed out in the bathroom and hit his head on the toilet.

"I think perhaps we can transfer your father to our skilled nursing unit for some rehabilitation," the doctor says. I say it all the time. Family members are uncertain what this means except that they don't have to take Dad home just yet and are temporarily grateful. The doctor has postponed answering the "What are we going to do with Dad?" question for a while longer. Every Medicare patient has coverage for one hundred lifetime SNU days if the criteria outlined in thousands of pages of regulations are met. But past the first week or two or three, these criteria usually can no longer be satisfied—not because the patient is well; very few get well once they get to the SNU—but because the patient is "no longer making progress." The patient is caught in the downward spiral of old age, disability, and dementia.

From here there is no "progress" except toward the grave. And the next way station is chronic custodial nursing home care. Family members will soon discover, if they haven't already, this essential Medicare insurance coverage fact: There is no Medicare coverage for long-term custodial nursing home care. Unless, of course, an elderly loved one is destitute, in which case he might qualify for some state-sponsored Medicaid assistance. And this often can be quite problematic, depending on the level at which his state reimburses its long-term care facilities.

And, typical of our government, as SNUs are being used more and more (as so many medical practitioners find themselves stymied by the "what are we going to do next?" question), Medicare has cut the reimbursements to these units drastically (not limiting the benefit to the patient, of course, which might anger the consuming public), so that many are closing. My own unit shrank to half its size before being shut down by its sponsoring hospital—even as I was writing this piece. Although the CEO told me that this was done because my hospital needed more "acute care beds"—certainly true—closing the SNU coincided with the change in Medicare reimbursements to SNUs that made it financially advantageous for acute care hospitals to jettison their SNUs in favor of more acute care beds.

The Road to Now

Thirty years ago I became a physician. My father, a first-generation American born of immigrant Russian Jews, was then the age I am now. He never completed high school. He was a sensitive man, who helped his fatherless family eke out a living through the Depression and then served five years in the Army Air Corps—a member of the "Greatest Generation." He ended up a man who was neither secure nor successful, even in this country's most optimistic years. But he was proud of me, a college boy, a medical school graduate.

In my family there was no more honorable profession than medicine, and the highest calling to my generation of physicians was the discipline of internal medicine—to follow in the footsteps of Sir William Osler, an empathic bedside clinician, a skilled diagnostician of the first order; to become a physician who derives great joy from shepherding his practice, his flock of interconnected families and friends through their medical lives, available for those frightening calls in the night, those tense moments in the ER, those difficult days in the intensive care unit (ICU); to be the one who is trusted to help make the tough choices, the final decisions, the one true patient advocate with broad knowledge, compassion, and unbiased judgment. More than half of the graduates of my medical school class pursued a career in general internal medicine. By 2003, that career choice among all first-year residents had declined to 19 percent.

Primary care, especially geriatric primary care, is time-consuming, excruciatingly detail-oriented professional piecework—all of those visits, those slowly moving, wheelchair-bound, unsteady elders to get onto and off of examination tables. Their pencil-scrawled complaints and medication lists to decipher, to question, to strip down, remake, and remodel at every encounter—a tiny dosage change here, an elimination or substitution there— all the time wondering: What am I missing? What else can I do? Not many young doctors want to preside over this carnage of human obsolescence or be reminded every working day of their own inevitable slide into disability and dementia.

In this work, the arenas change but not the inevitabilities: hospitals after the falls and broken hips; ICUs after the inevitable cascading complications of postoperative strokes, infections, and embolisms. Then the SNU and rehabilitation hospital admissions and, finally, custodial nursing homes. The patients become less responsive, less the people they used to be; their families become more uncertain, more demanding, more shrill from half a continent away. They call, fax, e-mail, wanting details, updates, help, answers. Visit by visit, I document declines. After a lifetime of practice, I find myself presiding over legions of chronically ill people—my extended family now— and every week there is another death certificate to sign, another condolence card to send, another funeral to attend.

There are many sexy career choices in medicine today, all the highly paid specialties and their procedures that actually—if all goes well—restore functioning and stave off death and disability, at least for a while. Snap in new knees or hips or shoulders. Laser the grunge out of blocked coronaries. Snip out the polyps that might become cancers. Suck out the fat, prop up the sags, botox the wrinkles, burn up the spider veins, pop in the new lenses, pump up the withered penis. Resolve the problem at hand, pocket the Medicare payment (or, even better, collect the full retail fee from "uncovered" procedures from your well-heeled patients), tell yourself what a great physician you are, and send your satisfied medical consumers back to their "primary geriatrician" quickly—before they fall, seize, stroke, and become incontinent on the plush-pile carpet of your waiting room.

Hospital Dangers

Three years ago my father, a longtime heart patient, had trouble breathing and complained of chest pain. He was admitted into the hospital with congestive heart failure. This is the hospital in which I have made rounds almost every day for the past three decades. Many of the nurses and therapists and I call each other by our first names. The CEO is my friend and patient. My father's physician is one of my young associates, well-trained and eager. I was confident that my father would receive the best medical care he could get in America today. Yet I would not leave him alone in his hospital room. During the day, if I or my brother or mother could not be there, I had a hired sitter by his bed.

It's rarely talked about, but acute hospitalizations are the most dangerous times for the elderly. Even if they have never before manifested any signs of confusion or disorientation, it is in the hospital—in a new and strange and threatening environment, under the influence of anesthetics, pain pills, antiemetics, and soporifics—where the elderly (competent or not) will meet their match. Add to this the iatrogenic mishaps (caused by the "normally expected" side effects and complications of standard medical procedures) and the human errors (mistakes in drug dosing, the right medication given to the wrong patient)—now multiplying in our modern hospitals like germs in a Petri dish—and it is almost a miracle that any elderly patient gets out of the hospital today relatively unscathed.

I stayed with my father every night; I slept in the reclining chair by his bed. I got up when he did; ran interference with bedrails, side tables, and IV poles; guarded his every move to the bathroom; looked at every medication that was handed to him and every fluid-filled bag plugged into his arm. I was not afraid to question the nurse or even call his physician. Each day my father descended deeper and deeper into paranoid confusion. He couldn't rest; he was intermittently unsure of who I was. At first I could calm him with my voice, talking about the old days, reminding him of our fishing trips on the Chesapeake Bay when I was young. Then he needed the physical reassurance of my hand on his arm or shoulder at all times. Finally, so that he could get some rest, I got in the bed with him and held him, comforting him as he once—in a long-ago life—did for me.

After four days and nights in the hospital, I knew I had to get my father out of there. His doctor came by and told me that his heart failure was better and that his dementia evaluation did not show a treatable or reversible cause. But he didn't like the way my father looked—he was agitated and sleep-deprived and deconditioned, a perfect candidate for some time in the SNU. And after all, here I was, his senior associate, the medical director of the SNU. Surely my dad would get good care there.

I took my father home. I knew if I didn't get him home at that moment, he would never come home again. The SNU for my dad would have been only a way station to a custodial nursing home. I arranged for a home health agency to come to my parents' house and provide my father with physical therapy to aid in his reconditioning and to assist with his bathing and dressing and grooming—something Medicare covers, but for only a limited period. I went to the pharmacy and filled the eight prescriptions he left the hospital with, and I went back again to buy the blue plastic container divided into daily dosing compartments when I realized that my mother was having trouble reading the labels on the bottles and following the instructions. How long had this been going on?

And Now We Wait

When I visit my father these days, if he is not asleep, I sit down beside him on the couch and talk at high volume into his hearing aid, if he has remembered it. Our conversations go something like this:

"How are you feeling today, Dad?"

"Not so good. You ought to come around more often."

"Dad, I was just here yesterday."

"Why are you calling me that? You're not my son."

"Of course I'm your son. That's your wife, my mother, sitting over there." (My mother: "What are you saying! Of course he's your son!")

"I like you and all, but you're not my son."

"Well, I love you anyway."

"You're older than I am. How could you be my son?"

"I love you, Dad."

"You ought to come around more often."

(My mother: "See what I'm putting up with all the time?")

Yet through the fog of his senility I still recognize my father, and once in a while he will surprise me. "Remember those big rockfish we used to catch off Thomas Point Light?" he might say. And then nothing.

The Medicare coverage for the home health care ran out almost as soon as it began. Between my brother and me, one of us is there almost every day. We have been fortunate to find two dedicated women to help my mother attend to my father's daily personal needs. My brother and I help with the cost of this care, which though considerable, is still less than the cost of custodial nursing home care. I often wonder: Why isn't this kind of care covered by Medicare or Medicaid? After all, when my parents use up their meager savings (which they will), like most families with a demented elder, they will become eligible for Medicaid, and the state will then pay the entire cost of custodial nursing home care. But the longer we can keep my father at home attended by aides, the cheaper his long-term care cost will be to society as a whole.

Drinking the supplemental nutritional feedings my brother brings to the house by the case (another noncovered cost of several hundred dollars a month), my father has actually put on a few pounds. I keep his medicines stocked, and I fiddle with the doses now and then, a tad extra diuretic when I see he is more short of breath, a tiny dose of an antipsychotic when he becomes more agitated. We get him in to see his doctor regularly for follow-up examinations and laboratory testing. And still, every week he gets worse, harder to deal with, more bizarre.

Recently, he has begun to holler at my mother every time she tries to help him change his clothes, which is often because he wets himself. "You're my sister! You're not supposed to see me naked!" he screams at her. He can no longer find his way from the living room to his bedroom in their tiny one-story house.

Most of us do not recognize when the mental capacities of our spouses or parents are reduced until something happens, something unexpected. My mother just didn't get it that my father was demented; she continued to believe his stubbornness and withdrawal were purposeful acts of belligerence against her. Until the day she realized he could no longer figure out how to unlock the front door by himself, she continued to blame him for his disability. Adult children are often no different in their lack of insight; we expect our parents, after all, to be our parents. Dad is just being cold and distant because he's still angry over something from years before, a son might believe. The sad fact is that Dad forgot about this incident long, long ago.

From my years as a geriatrician and now as the son of an "old old" man, I recognize that there is but one inescapable truth: Our parents will become our children if they live long enough. Perhaps if we looked on our elderly in this way, we would be kinder to them. They will become dependent on us, our stronger arms, our acts of gentleness and caring. We will arrange for their meals, pay their bills, take them to their doctor visits, sit by their bedsides at the hospital and in the nursing home.

I don't know what else to do for Dad at this moment, but I know what is likely to happen to him if he does not die in his sleep, a heaven-sent coup de grâce that from long experience I recognize is unlikely to occur. There is almost always a great struggle in the end. One day I will get a frantic call from my mother that he is on the floor and she cannot get him up, and he is crying out in terrible pain. Wherever I am, I will drop what I am doing and race over there and find that one of his legs is shortened and externally rotated. His hip is broken. From the wall phone in my parents' kitchen, I will call my brother and I will tell him all the reasons why we should not send him to the hospital: He might not recover from the surgery—indeed, might die on the table given his bad heart. But even if he does survive, he will spend days in the ICU, probably on a respirator, until his heart is stable. And then he will be constantly confused and agitated. I don't see him ever being able to cooperate with physical therapy. At best he will end up in a nursing home, bedridden and at the mercy of overworked, underpaid aides. He will descend deeper and deeper into disorientation and delusion, require medications to keep him from harming himself, and die anyway in a few months—or perhaps even a year or two if he is unfortunate and the care is better than average.

My brother will hear my mother crying and my father hollering in the background. He will feel guilty that he is not in the house with me at that moment. He will remember the time our father took us on a summer vacation to the White Face Mountains and we all huddled together on the swinging bridge in the mist, as the Ausable River tumbled and roared through High Falls Gorge. Then he will say, "Maybe it won't be as bad as you think. Maybe we can set up a hospital bed in his room—I think the door is wide enough—and it won't take much to alter the shower to accommodate a wheelchair." There will be a moment of silence. "I don't know," he'll say. "You're the doctor. What do you think we should do?"

I do not tell him that I often, in fitful sleep, dream that when the time comes I go to my father's bedside, quietly fill a syringe with morphine, and stroke his arm as I place the tourniquet. I tell him over and over again how much I love him and what a good father he has been to me as I slip the needle into his antecubital vein. Then I say how much I will miss him and goodbye, Dad, goodbye, as I push the contents into his bloodstream. In this dream I tell my mother and my brother that he has gone peacefully in his sleep.

Yet I have not until now given voice to this dream because I know for certain that in the end, I could never do this. Not to my poor, demented, suffering father. Not to anyone. I know there are some who disagree with me, and perhaps this is one way our society will ultimately deal with its flood of elders in this age of limits. I will by then, I hope, be old and no longer on the front lines. When my time comes—before it comes—I will choose for myself. But for now, as long as I have the will and the strength to practice, I am a physician deeply steeped and firmly rooted in the art and tradition of healing, of comforting.

For my father, on that day, I will tell my brother that I will handle it and hang up the phone. Then I'll pick it up again and dial 911.

∽ Kidneys and the Kindness of Strangers

A medical ethicist changes his mind about altruistic donors.

DAVID STEINBERG

One day a patient of ours with end-stage kidney failure asked whether, if he found a stranger willing to give him a kidney, our surgeons would retrieve and transplant the organ. The man posing the question required dialysis and could anticipate a wait of several years before receiving a kidney transplant. The question was then presented by our

Volume 22, Number 4. July/August 2003. This work was supported by a grant from the Karp Family Foundation in memory of Harold Karp.

kidney transplant team to the medical ethics group that I head at a hospital in a small town thirteen miles northwest of Boston.

The patient's request was unusual; it was made after the patient read about a thirty-six-year-old woman from Texas who through the Internet found a stranger willing to give her a kidney. The transplant team wanted to know: Would honoring this request be morally appropriate? Thus began my own search into the implications of kidney donation by altruistic strangers.

Clarifying Motives

I found Susan by chance when searching for "altruistic donors" on Google. Her note said that she wanted to give one of her kidneys free to someone who needed one. I wrote to her because I was curious about her motives. It seemed bizarre to me to submit to the risks and discomforts of surgery in order to help a total stranger. And, as a medical ethicist, I knew that not every altruistic act is necessarily a "good" act. Donating a kidney is not risk-free. If a donor dies, the morality of such a donation could be called into doubt.

Through e-mail conversations with Susan, I probed and questioned to unearth the personality or cognitive defect that I assumed would explain her reckless altruism. I ended up, however, wondering whether, of the two of us, she was the more rational. Part of our e-mail dialogue, edited for clarity, went like this.

> ME: I am interested in learning why someone would donate a kidney to a stranger.
>
> SUSAN: I believe I should try to help people. This seems to be a perfect opportunity to help someone in a big way with minimal inconvenience to myself. You may think 'minimal' is a strange word to use regarding a kidney transplant. However, I understand the laparoscopic surgery is very good and I should recover in about a month. Do you need a kidney?
>
> ME: No, I don't. Are you aware that there is a small but real possibility of death—perhaps one in 2,500—if you donate your kidney?
>
> SUSAN: When I first thought about giving a kidney, I was a bit freaked out thinking about the worst-case scenario—death or rejection by the other person of my kidney. I guess that's where my faith in God comes into it. I believe God wants me to use my life to help other people, and

the rewards will be a much deeper happiness and a sense of real ful-
fillment in my life. Many people are willing to *kill* for what they believe in; why not allow people who are willing to take personal risks do
what they believe in to *save* a life? Anyway, a one in 2,500 chance of
death is a pretty slim one. Part of the skepticism people feel about my
decision is that the subject of live organ transplants is relatively new and
still controversial. People need time to think through the issues and get
over their initial reaction, which is usually based on ignorance and
fear.

At first my conversations with Susan were impersonal; gradually I learned
a few things about her. At the end of one note she signed her full name, Susan Gianstefani. She told me that she was an Australian citizen living in London with her husband and that she stayed at home to tutor her seven-year-
old son.

Unusual But Firm Beliefs

Susan's altruism is rare; donation by altruistic strangers makes up less than 1
percent of live kidney donations in the United States. Most live organ transplants take place between people who have an established relationship. Live
kidney donations have become more common than those from deceased
donors and produce better outcomes. But they are questionable because
they place healthy people at risk, a situation that is incompatible with medicine's traditional goals. I persisted in questioning Susan's motives.

> ME: Most people who believe in God do not donate a kidney to a stranger.
> Are there experiences in your life that explain why you have decided
> to do this? Are you acting out of guilt?
> SUSAN: Just because "most" people don't do it, isn't a reason to ban the mi-
> nority who want to donate to a stranger. Of course there are experi-
> ences that have influenced my decision to donate. I have given blood
> for many years, so the idea of giving something from my body is not
> new to me. I am on the donor list for bone marrow transplants. I have
> learned that showing love to others makes me happy as well as the per-
> son I am loving! I feel sad that I only have one spare kidney! It's true
> that I feel guilty about some things. However, I am not trying to "pay

back" God because of guilt. I believe God has forgiven me for the bad things I have done.

ME: Did you consider that if anything went wrong, your seven-year-old son would not have a mother?

SUSAN: Yes, but that shouldn't make me the sort of person who locks herself away fearing something bad will happen. People take all sorts of risks as parents. What about police and firemen? Should they be told they shouldn't do their jobs because if something happens to them their children will have one less parent? They choose to take a risk for the sake of the good that they are achieving through their dangerous occupations. If I am willing to take some risks to help others, overall my life will be a lot better than a pathetic existence of fear and self-preservation. Also, if I don't donate my kidney to someone, maybe their children will lose a parent or have a parent living on dialysis. The best I can do for my son as a mother is give him a good example. If I die, he will still have a loving, dedicated father, which is more than a lot of other children have.

Skirting the Law to Do Good

Susan held some surprises, revealed when I asked her if there was anything else she wanted me to know. "So far, I have two potential recipients," she wrote. "One, George, is from Colorado, and the other is a woman from Scotland. I chose them because we share the same blood group and they were the first to contact me. This week I will be sending blood samples to the USA to confirm that I match with George. It will be interesting to see what happens when I arrive at the hospital with instructions on obtaining blood samples. You see, it is illegal in the UK for me to donate my kidney without going through a regulatory body to determine that I am doing it for a 'close friend.'"

Surprise number one—Susan was performing an illegal act. In the United Kingdom, organ donation to someone other than one of a specified category of genetic relatives requires approval of the Unrelated Live Transplant Regulatory Authority, which requires information about the relationship between donor and recipient and documentary evidence, such as a copy of a marriage certificate or family photographs, substantiating the relationship. (Organ donation by strangers is also prohibited in other countries, including Germany and India.) Susan's kidney donation to a stranger was going to violate British law. "Donating my kidney to someone over the Internet is not the best way to do it," Susan wrote. "I believe the best way is to go through a hospital; however, because of the laws here, I cannot use those channels."

Susan's second surprise came in an e-mail from Jon Ronson, a documentary filmmaker in London. Susan had given me permission to use our e-mail conversations at a Harvard Medical School ethics conference, where I planned to tell her story and stimulate discussion of organ donation by altruistic strangers. Ronson wanted to film the conference because he was making a documentary of Susan's illegal (in her country) attempt to become an altruistic kidney donor to a stranger.

I sensed that I had at last uncovered the elusive flaw that explained Susan's motivation. As tactfully as possible, I asked if she wasn't simply a crusader looking for publicity. "I should have mentioned Jon's interest earlier, but I didn't want media interest to cloud the issues," she responded. "I expect some people will doubt my intentions are genuine. The publicity, although it will make more people aware of the issues, will also be a convenient way to disregard the real motivation of someone altruistically donating an organ out of love. It is human nature to be skeptical. I hope some people will appreciate there aren't many people who would give a kidney to a stranger simply to get publicity. There isn't much I can do to prove my true motives. However, since Jon Ronson is going to make this documentary, I feel excited about inspiring others to donate their kidneys altruistically."

At this point I realized that Susan was genuine. I conceded that human brains are wired differently and that for some of us, donating an organ to a stranger seems an appropriate and natural response.

Having Faith

Susan waited a long time before telling me about the Jesus Christians. "I am also part of a small group of believers who actively try to get people thinking about doing things for love rather than for selfish reasons," she wrote. "Quite a few of us have decided to donate our kidneys to strangers for free, because this fits what the Bible teaches about healing the sick, those who have two giving to those who have none, etc. Two of us have donated through a hospital already and are recovering well. We have been living and working as a community for over twenty years. We are called Jesus Christians. You can check our Web site, www.jesuschristians.com. We are a 'church' in the sense that we are a group of believers in Jesus and his teachings. The worldwide population of the group is only about twenty-five people; more than half are here in London, and the others are in Texas, India, and Australia. Almost half of us are interested in donating a kidney to a stranger; we have kept our kidney donations secret from the public in general (with reference to our community) to avoid the anticipated media frenzy we think may accompany such an action by a group of people."

Was Susan an independent thinker who was a member of a like-minded group, or was she an intelligent but brain-washed member of a cult? "The fact that you belong to a group will serve as a red flag and make people wonder whether you have been subtly and subconsciously manipulated by the group," I wrote. "I suppose an analogy might be the hundreds of people who committed suicide in Jonestown."

She got angry. "I felt offended and disappointed by the comments in your last letter," Susan wrote. "The fact that you are a 'doctor' made me want to give you more time and respect. However, given that you probably would not even consider donating a kidney to a stranger, I can't help feeling you should respect the group I belong to. Yet it seems the opposite is true. You and other doctors have set yourselves up as judges of our motives with the possible intention of preventing hospitals from accepting the gift of our kidneys."

I didn't want our conversation to end; I apologized to Susan and later asked again, "Were you exposed to any group pressure to donate?"

"No," she answered. "We are all very aware that this is a decision that cannot and should not be made lightly, and if anyone donates under any sort of pressure from others in the community, that would be wrong."

Susan's reasons for donating a kidney were rational and consistent with her religious beliefs; she could anticipate happiness as a reward for her altruism. Despite my reservation that we should always feel some discomfort at removing a kidney from a healthy person, my e-mail discussion with Susan convinced me that in carefully selected cases, using guidelines that adequately protect donors, it is morally appropriate for some people to donate a kidney to someone they don't know. My conversations with Susan also made me realize that altruistic donors' highly developed sense of solidarity with humankind should prod the rest of us. We should be embarrassed that the altruistic stranger suffers and accepts risk to donate an organ, while most of us have not even filled out an organ donor card to permit retrieval of our organs after we die.

A Better System

More than 50,000 people in the United States are waiting for a kidney. In 2001, 2,834 people died while on the waiting list. Our current system has failed to meet demand. We cannot legislate altruism, and there are few Susans in the world. We can, however, promote enlightened self-interest.

When we are young and healthy, and it is unknown who will need a kidney and who will die and be eligible to donate one, we should be given the opportunity to opt in as "organ donors." An organ donor whose fate is to need a kidney would receive preferential treatment. This system would produce more organ donors because it would become advantageous to be an organ donor. Healthy people who already have signed organ donor cards voluntarily under the present system would be permitted to join the new pool.

The system would at first apply only to donations from deceased donors, to avoid practical problems such as live donors who change their minds after reaping the benefits of being in the pool. This approach would bring the supply of kidneys from deceased donors closer to demand while also eliminating the unfairness of the organ taker–organ giver divide. People needing organs other than kidneys could also benefit because deceased donors can donate all salvageable organs. Government support of a central registry and legislation to prohibit reneging by the next of kin would be needed. Countries such as Belgium and Spain have adopted a similar approach, using a doctrine of "presumed consent" that permits organ retrieval unless an individual has specifically opted out.

Susan—one of those rare people who do not need the spur of enlightened self-interest to donate an organ—called me when she arrived in the United States. It was the first time we had spoken. I asked her if she was nervous about her operation. She said she was excited. I spoke with her again after her surgery at the University of Wisconsin. All went well. She met and liked George, the recipient of her kidney, whom she affectionately described as a "character." Despite some discomfort, she was in good spirits.

Susan had changed my mind about altruistic kidney donations. To my great surprise, through my acquaintance with her I could respond in the affirmative to the transplant team's query about the morality of a kidney transplant from an appropriate altruistic stranger.

⁓ The Curtain

What happens when doctors reach out to bereaved family members.

W. Richard Boyte

Churches are well-known local landmarks in rural Mississippi. They are the location for so many central events of small-town life: worship, family reunions, baptisms, town meetings, elections, weddings, and funerals. So I was not surprised to get detailed directions to my young patient's church from the smiling convenience store clerk. Nevertheless, I worried that I would be late as I drove down one and then another narrow two-lane road.

Circumstances had not allowed me much time to drive to this small town in the southern region of the state. That morning, as I supervised patient rounds with residents assigned to the pediatric intensive care unit (PICU), I had felt anxious and rushed. My duties as a PICU attending physician at a children's hospital that afternoon were graciously being covered by one of my partners. Now, as I pulled into a gravel parking lot on that cool, windy Saturday afternoon in March, I was relieved to see that I was among the first to arrive.

I sat for a moment in the car and searched the faces of the small group of African Americans gathering at the front of the simple wooden building. I did not recognize anyone. Disappointed, I left the car and made my way to the front entrance. I quickly walked to one of several wooden straight-back pews at the back. Seated, I glanced around nervously. The unassuming sanctuary painted in shades of white and gray was quiet except for the sounds of

Volume 21, Number 4: 242–245. July/August 2002.

children playing outside. Sunlight shone through windows on either side, attempting to brighten the room. Slowly, people drifted in to sparsely fill the pews.

As I considered the small likelihood that I would blend unnoticed into this unfamiliar setting, my thoughts naturally drifted to Sherri. The memories of her beaming face and toothy smile failed to comfort me. "Oh God," I whispered out loud, "I still can't believe it." Just then a side door at the front of the sanctuary opened. Through the opening a group of men in dark suits entered solemnly, escorting a small coffin. They placed it in front of the altar. Sherri's family filed in slowly to be seated in the front pews.

I had never before attended the funeral of a patient. I was always concerned that my presence would somehow add to the grief of parents and family members. But I felt compelled to attend this funeral because of my relationship with Sherri. After all, I had known her for half of her nearly nine-year life.

Knowing Sherri

I met Sherri almost five years earlier when she was afflicted with a devastating pneumonia. Sickle cell anemia made her more susceptible to serious infection and lung disease. Complications from her illness would threaten her life over the days and weeks that followed her admission to the PICU. Because her condition hid her true self, I came to know her initially through her parents and grandparents. Their love for this child was pure and boundless. My respect for her family grew as I witnessed their courage under the most straining of life's trials. No one should ever face the possibility of losing a child. More than once I told them that the chance for her surviving was very small.

In large part due to grace, she did survive. Her recovery, however, would be a long and laborious process. She was left in a weakened state and would require the continued assistance of a mechanical ventilator. Over that time, I observed this child bravely pull the scattered pieces of her person back together. She was soon demonstrating the intelligence, humor, and curiosity that her family had described so well. After a while she was finally freed from mechanical ventilation.

I looked forward to the moments we could share. She could make me smile during even the worst of my busy days. She became a relentless chatterbox who called out to me whenever I was present in the PICU. We would spend whatever minutes I could spare reading children's books, watching videos, or playing board games. She was eventually transferred from the PICU to a wardroom.

Her long hospitalization continued under the supervision of a different pediatrician, but I tried to visit her often. Sometimes, however, she did not feel it was often enough. After a short absence on my part, I visited, only to find her ignoring me.

"Aren't you going to say hello?" I asked.

"To who?" she replied.

"To me," I answered, somewhat hurt.

"Oh," she said with dramatized indifference, "I'm not sure I know you. Do you work here?"

In the years that followed her discharge, I would see her nearly every month on her outpatient visits to the hematology clinic. Either her mother would bring her to my office or I would go to her. On her visits to my office she would look about until she spied something, usually a small knick-knack from the bookshelf, to occupy her attention. Without fail, she would ask to take it home. I began to keep small gifts for her in my office. Despite all her earlier difficulties, once again she was able to resume her life as a busy, bright, and happy child.

I remember our last morning together in sharp detail. It was about five a.m. when the phone rang. This is not an unusual occurrence when I am taking call. The resident in the PICU was dutifully reporting to me his most recent admission. His description of an eight-year-old girl experiencing respiratory distress was, at first, nothing highly out of the ordinary. Then he mentioned her name. Cursing softly, I sat upright in bed. "Do you know her?" he asked. After a long pause I answered, "Yes, I know her."

When I arrived, she looked deeply asleep. Her chest rose and fell in rapid, labored breaths. Her face was partially hidden behind an oxygen mask. I touched her shoulder and was surprised when she opened her eyes. She whispered a weak hello. "You're going to be all right," I said. She nodded slowly and closed her eyes again. I then listened to her lungs and reviewed her lab work. Her nurse told me that her mother and grandparents were in the family waiting room. I found them and told them that she would again require the ventilator.

Sherri's dark brown eyes opened wide when I told her about the ventilator. For us to place a tube in her trachea for mechanical ventilation, she would need to be sedated. I explained to her that I would give her medicine to make her sleep and that she would be kept asleep until she was better. Her eyes searched mine carefully. "When will I wake up?" she asked. I was stunned by her question. After a moment of uncomfortable silence I answered, "I don't know, honey. Soon, I hope."

She never did awaken. Her diseased lungs did not respond to support from mechanical ventilation or any of our other efforts. Later that morning, I was forced to say goodbye.

Erecting the Barricade

The minister delivered a passionate sermon and eulogy, but my thoughts began to wander. I began to think of Sherri's last moments and those of other children who had been my patients. I have been a witness to the circumstances and consequences of death all too often. Long ago I found my curtain. Like so many of my colleagues, I have learned to pull it closed at times of death. I have done so to protect myself.

As a medical student, I had my first glimpse of the curtain. I was standing against a wall, nervously witnessing a resuscitation for the first time. The patient was not expected by his physician to survive. The code team was working feverishly but somewhat mechanically through the appropriate protocol. Just outside the room, the patient's friends and family members anxiously awaited the outcome. Inside the room, the code team members joked with each other and, between tasks, animatedly discussed a variety of subjects. But then, each time a team member left the room, it was as if an invisible curtain had to be pulled aside. On one side of the curtain were lighthearted jokes and camaraderie. On the other side, as bad news was broken, faces were held in serious expressions.

Formal bereavement training for physicians is rare. Example becomes the teacher in this void. I was taught to use the curtain by example, and I have learned to carry it with me. I have seen it in others, who I assume were taught in the same manner. As a physician, I am somehow supposed to rise above the emotional impact of death. I am a professional. I am touched, outraged, saddened, guilt-ridden, and horrified, but I am able to place my emotions behind the curtain. There, others will not see them. Perhaps I will not experience them as strongly. Perhaps I will not feel them at all. I have been taught indirectly that this is a duty. Humor, however inappropriate, often helps to keep the curtain closed.

When Doctors Turn Off Their Humanity

My own use of the curtain began to change early in my residency training when my father died. This was well before I fully understood the curtain. I recall hearing laughter come from the physicians' station in the cardiac intensive care unit. At that tremendously painful moment in my life, how could anyone be experiencing joy? I resented it deeply.

Since then I have seen that the curtain can be harmful. Too often it is a barrier to communication. We physicians don't know what is appropriate to say when we ourselves don't know how we feel. We sometimes do not communicate at all. Even when there is nothing to put into words, we miss the opportunity to be supportive with our presence. We cheat our patients, their loved ones, and ourselves. At death there may not be anything I can say or do to lighten the burden of the bereaved. But there are so many ways my actions might add to the weight.

More and more often I have pulled the curtain open. In so doing, I have become a better physician. My clinical skills may not have changed, but my capacity for compassion has grown along with my ability to understand and experience the human condition. This was brought home to me the night I met the grandmother of an infant dying from complications of meningitis. I was leaving the baby's room at the time. Knowing nothing more could be done medically, I expressed my regrets to the baby's grandmother. When she thanked me anyway, I tried to deflect her gratitude. I told her that I wished I could have done more. She shook her head and said, "No, I am thanking you for your tears."

To attend Sherri's funeral, I had to pull open the curtain. I knew that by doing so I would be vulnerable to the elements of grief and would experience the ravages of emotion. Indeed, I felt intense sorrow, loss, anger, and frustration. But I also realized that her family's pain and grief were much greater than mine could ever be. As I stood with the other mourners at the graveside for the minister's final prayer, I again worried that my presence would be seen as an intrusion.

Afterward, her parents and grandparents approached me. In her mother's hands was an item from one of the floral arrangements: a toy cloth rabbit dressed as an angel. With a tearful smile she presented it to me as a gift. It greets me every morning from my dresser, reminding me to keep the curtain open as far as I can.

INDEX